the big and me

Paul Doody

Published in 2020 by Eddie Doody

ISBN:

A CIP catalogue copy of this book can be found in the British Library.

Published with the help of Indie Authors World
www.indieauthorsworld.com

IndieAuthors
World

All statistics are quoted from www.nhsconfed.org and are
correct for England and Wales as of May 2013

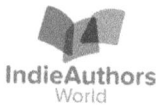

To Steven: wherever you've gone and wherever we might go

Contents

My NHS

In August 2012 a ticking time bomb literally blew up in my lap. "the big C". I had been given a diagnosis of bladder cancer and needed a long course of treatment and radical surgery if I wanted to see much more than my 42 years. My likelihood of developing this type of cancer was extremely low but here it was: rare, life-threatening and utterly compelling.

A cancer diagnosis is momentous and given by medicine to one in three of us, over the course of a lifetime. Cancer rates are on the increase and yet rates of survival are better now than at any time in human history. So why do we all worry if the statistics are so positive? For most it's the treatment for cancer that carries the greatest worry.

Even though the treatment is safe, accurate and proven effective, it scares the hell out of the newly diagnosed and their families. Just the thought of the regime; the sickness, the baldness, the surgery and with no guarantee of success, it's enough to bring the strongest of us to our knees. My NHS though has exceptional rates of early diagnosis and intervention.

The National Health Service was brought into being in 1948, based on the Beveridge Report (1942) to create "comprehensive health and rehabilitation services for prevention and cure of disease". It was to be funded entirely through taxation, allowing access regardless of income.

Health Secretary Aneurin Bevan opened ParkHospital in Manchester on July 5th and in doing so created the world's first centrally funded health care system. It's my NHS (and yours) and even to this day there's nothing quite like it anywhere else in the world.

Treatment is free at the point of care and all decisions made by the organisation are based on the best clinical outcome. This point is pivotal to the NHS (and it's a huge point) but seldom appreciated for what it means. I had worked in the NHS since 1989 and fully endorsed that my patients would receive the best care and equipment available from me but personally I had never needed significant care from my parent employer.

Recently, using an online health calculator, I estimated that the cost of my own treatment over eight months had been approximately £120,000 or roughly three times my gross annual salary. The total NHS expenditure for the year 2012 / 2013 amounted to £106.6 billion. That may seem like a lot.

However thinking about my own numbers in a little detail, based on my monthly salary contributions alone, it would take me 444 months to pay that back. That is roughly 37 years at my current wage to offset what I have used in resources from the Health Service. This is all in a relatively short time frame.

My care has been decided by my Consultants on best practice and greatest life expectancy. If I lived in the USA for example, my health care provider would be deciding on behalf of my clinicians "the best cost effectiveness" of my treatment. Think about the differences on offer between the two systems. Cost effective is still a tenet in the NHS (and always has been) but the other system employs a value bias and can overrule *any* clinician's decision which has been based on the outcome (survival is what we're ultimately talking about here).

The Commonwealth Fund in 2010 compared six other countries' health care systems. (Australia, Canada, the Netherlands, USA, Germany and New Zealand) The NHS was rated best system in terms of efficiency, effective care and cost-related problems. It was ranked second overall and second for equity and safe care.

The NHS has its flaws as all man made things do but it strives for constant improvement. The humans within the organisation make rare mistakes but systems are already in place so that we learn from them. The NHS steadily evolves and adapts to new technology and therapies. It is driven to treat all its patients in a safe, accurate and effective way.

The NHS deals with over one million patients every 36 hours.

It's my NHS and I won't hear a bad word against it.

A Crap Birthday

I spent my 43rd birthday in unfamiliar surroundings; being prodded by strangers and wondering if my luck had truly run out. Needless to say I'd had better celebrations. Poor health, poor timing and irony had conspired to make this a memorable date for all the wrong reasons.

Gartnavel General Hospital, 5th of February 2013. 9am the day before my cancer operation wasn't the venue for an ad-hoc party. Nor was there any cake, banners, cards or gifts. Turning up to this particularly unattractive edifice so early in the morning gave me an impression of voluntarily signing into prison. Built 42 years ago, it is a grey, eight storey brick testament to bad 70s architecture.

The impression of incarceration isn't helped by the chain link attached to its frontage. This has nothing whatsoever to do with keeping the inmates (patients) in but simply to stop birds roosting and crapping over the window ledges. I had seen the building many times before, having worked here for years but on this particular morning I was seeing it in a whole different light.

This was, hopefully, the final instalment in a whirlwind of diagnosis and treatment that had been going on for months and months. I still wished there were some candles to blow out.

What there was, oh lucky me, was 4 litres of bowel prep to get through before 11pm. Anyone not familiar with this cleansing fluid pre-op should imagine a salty, cloudy, briny foul mix which I imagine is as palatable as licking a fisherman's arse. I had to choke this stuff down regularly throughout the day whilst humming "happy birthday to me." It was grim.

I was in a four bedded room with only two other occupants. Neither was particularly effusive; one guy was attached to a drip and sat the whole day staring vacantly into space. The other slept solidly throughout the day pausing occasionally to let out some serious farts before turning over and resuming his sack time.

Our room was a curious mix of old and new. The bed was a fully electric modern masterpiece; multi position adjustable and ultra-high tech. The walls in contrast had old Formica panels and melamine electrical outlets. Each of the four bays had curtain tracks that looked as if they had been taken from a seventies sit-com.

The drip pump attached to one roommate was a new precision instrument delivering digital dosages of his prescription and yet the windows had seen so many coats of gloss paint you couldn't see the hinges. My two comrades seemed unaffected by the strange mix of past and future but truth be told they had very little to say despite my best efforts at banter.

No matter, I had Tom Clancy for company, having been given his latest hardback by my Dad. However just a couple of hours (and a couple of hundred pages) into my cocktail of gag inducing brine, something was beginning to happen.

At first it was a small gurgling sound down below. Then it was a noise like sink being emptied and then it was an "oh my god, get out of the way" dash to the loo. This was like nuclear fallout for your arse. This stuff could strip the lining from engines. At least that was it over for now. Or so I thought.

The whole rest of the day was an unrelenting rush to the toilet in a mad panic. Where was this all coming from? My two cohorts started using the convenience across the hall as I was monopolising ours so much. It got so bad I was taking Mr Clancy's book with me otherwise I was never going to get the bloody thing read. As birthdays go this was literally and figuratively crap. How the hell had I end up in this situation?

How I Ended up in This Situation

A family holiday in August 2012 was going splendidly. The family was comprised of Stephanie (wife), Arianne (10 year old daughter), Jonathan (8 year old son), Anne (Mother and Nan to the kids) and Eddie (Father and Papa to the kids).

Lincolnshire was green, flat, beautiful and warm. We'd all been here 2 years previously, in a log cabin by a lake and all agreed it was worthy of a second visit. Whilst the others were worrying about more mundane holiday related topics: at what point did the leisure centre open, how to fit in all the sights and most of all how to block out Eddie's goddamn snoring, I was worried about the alarming gouts of blood every time I went for a pee.

We're not talking a mild discolouration in the wee wee here. This was full on blood red; Beelzebub's own urinal. It had been going on for days but what's worse, I felt 100% fine. No pain, no burn, no urgency and no distress apart from the B movie special effects issuing from my knob.

This was no kidney infection; I'd had loads of those in my day. I'd inherited kidney stones from Anne. I was trying loads of water to flush things through; still no good. I started drinking tons of cranberry juice. So much in fact that people were beginning to wonder if I had cystitis. If it continued, I'd need to call in some favours once I got back to work. For the time being it was relax, enjoy the scenery and close my eyes tight each time I went to the loo.

At this point I'd worked in the NHS for 22 years as an Audiologist. You get to work one-on-one with someone with hearing, balance or tinnitus problems. Your environment is quiet, calm and most of the time you get to restore a most valuable sense to someone who ends up stunned and very grateful.

The Daily Telegraph in 2011 put it number 6 in the least stressful jobs to have (I'd argue strongly against that statistic in the modern NHS with 18 week targets, waiting times, quality standards, blah, blah). Computer software designer was number 1 in case you were wondering.

However, if job satisfaction is what you're after, then Audiology is an excellent patient centred, quality of life driven, scientific and therapeutic career. I love my job and happened to find one day that I was offered the head of department role in Glasgow Royal Infirmary. Bonus!

The actual bonus to 22 years in the NHS however is a wealth of contacts; friends who are willing to help at the drop of a hat if you've found something broken in your Willy. Karen at Spinal Injuries was my first call; I have been a paraplegic and in a wheelchair since age three, having run in front of a car, unaware of the "Green Cross Code" at that point. The folk at Spinal Injuries assess me once a year; just to make sure I'm not faking. I'm not, as far as they can tell.

Karen is a true friend and I made a begging call to ask for a hasty referral to be sent directly to me for a KUB, a Kidney, Ureter and Bladder scan, so I could take it to yet another friend in Radiology where I worked. The referral duly went to Audrey in CT at the Royal and within 4 days of being back at work I had my scans booked. All this could only have happened with the kindness of others. For those who work in the NHS, you still can rely on professional treatment from your friends.

The head of Radiology (yes, I received top notch professional treatment) was all sweetness and light and chatty like a host on talk radio, right up to the point she found something "weird" in the bladder. All pleasantries ended and she became business. Sizing, dimensions, locations and terminology only a select few understand was dictated into a machine. It could have been Chinese algebra equations for all I knew.

The words which stuck out were bladder and wart. Now to explain; medicine couches uncomfortable words and diagnoses in seemingly less threatening terminology. I wasn't being fooled by the "wart" euphemism. I knew fine well a bladder wart was a tumour. Tumour: there's a word which comes with a sinking feeling.

Yet more urgent investigating needed to be done. Now I had to find the best Urological surgeon by asking as many people in the know. Mr Fraser's name cropped up more than once. That was the name for me. All agreed he was "The Man" if your willy was wonky, so I begged the receptionist for the first available cancellation appointment, which I got (preferential treatment again).

Cool, calm and collected.

Me: not him. I wanted the facts in a bald manner, the baldest manner. Balder even, than Bruce Willis.

"Hit me".

He did. Bladder tumours can be muscle invasive or not. Grading is T1, T2 and T3. Everyone hopes for a nice easily removed surface T1, as it's opposite, a muscle invasive T3, has piss poor survivability. For piss poor read, 83% of people don't make it 5 years post op. Neither Mr Fraser nor I would know the grade until he did a TURBT. Trans Urethral Resection of Bladder Tumour: "Trans Urethral" yep, up the one eyed pipe with camera and cutter. I was so looking forward to this.

Stephanie wanted to know the minute I was out of the consultation but on reflection perhaps a text wasn't the best way to break the news. Just because I'm frank and fact biased doesn't mean everyone wants their news quite so stark.

At home time that evening I was busy tidying up the kid's dinner dishes when she got in from work. As she entered the kitchen I realised I'd made a huge mistake. Her eyes were red-rimmed and her usual flawless makeup was streaked and blotchy. We talked, we hugged and then she cried. Then she researched.

She researched a lot. Stephanie is the type of self-driven knowledge seeking Brainiac that I'm not. She is the Stephen Hawking type, needing research which is validated and peer reviewed. I'm the type that needs to know what needs done and then how much Top Gear I can fit in before it all kicks off. As far as I was concerned we knew nothing till after the TURBT so I wasn't going to tie my brain in knots with scary vague possibilities. I tried explaining this but I was just in the way of her flow charts and Venn diagrams. (I'm being glib purely for effect, you understand).

At this point I was plodding along in probable denial. I tried some light reading on medical journals but that was no good. They were awash with statistics of survivability versus age versus category. Some of the stats were super optimistic provided you fit into an early stage cancer and had quick surgery. Other survivability rates were so pessimistic you had a better chance of catching a thrown spear between your teeth.

The various cancer support websites were too touchy feely

for my tastes "We're there for you, every part of your journey." The kind of thing that makes my skin crawl with fake empathy. The sheer scope of what surgically could be done was remarkable but conversely some of the end results from surgery were horrific. There were lots of pictures. I stopped looking early on. In part it was because the categorising of my tumour hadn't been done but also because the web was scaring me shitless.

Too many variables were hanging in the air. There was no point in researching bladder cancer to the nth degree because where would you stop? Once we knew a little more, the internet could be used as an information source for all involved. I asked everyone who knew me not to go looking stuff up in the meantime, at least until we knew what we were up against. I was convincing no one, least of all myself. Besides, not one single person I knew listened to a single word I'd said.

Bastards!

TURBT

"Have you ever smoked?"
"No"
"Never, you're sure?"
"No, never"

This would be my most often repeated question and answer. Every medic, consultant, FY1, registrar, nurse, tea lady and porter asked the same damn thing, over and over. Apparently smoking and bladder cancer go like strawberries and cream, like Laurel and Hardy, like me and Top Gear.

"No", "No, never", "Nope", "Uh-Uh", "Negative", "No way, Jose' ". How many ways do you want me to say the same thing. I found it unbelievable that they had no way to link me with cancer. Medics hate it when it's "just one of those things" and most members of the public would throw a hissy fit at being told this. I had been around healthcare long enough to know better.

Being in a 'chair wasn't a risk factor, excess coffee drinking wasn't a risk factor (thank god for that, my coffee intake bordered on addiction), just as being an Aquarius or blue eyed wasn't a risk factor. Being increasingly frustrated with the same line of questioning though, was definitely a risk factor to the medic's health. Get on with it.

They got on with it. September's TURBT op was scheduled in Glasgow's Southern General hospital and I welcomed it with a spring in my step (in the absence of a wheelchair analogy). I was desperate for the "Cracking on" to see the end of this. It was comparatively easy surgery with a light general anaesthetic and only an hour or so under.

I was riding high on optimism. A nice easy, surface "wart" was my assumption. Once my surgeon had cauterised and removed the offending article I would be back at my desk a week or so later and life would continue on in its familiar routine.

On waking from the operation though Mr Fraser was there above me, hovering over the table. "How long have you had frank symptoms again?"

"Since August."

"No longer?"

"No."

"And you've never smoked cigarettes?" I tried to throw him my best sneer but with the remnants of a general anaesthetic in me, it probably looked more like a stroke.

"No!"

"Ok, I'll see you back in clinic in a couple of weeks." The post op couple of weeks dragged by very slowly. More so since I was nursing a knob that felt like it had been dipped in molten lava. The relative ease and speed of the operation was obviously due to the fact he was using surgical power tools sourced from B&Q (Block and Quayle were the founders in case you were wondering). This was very real pain in the area of a man's anatomy usually treated with the utmost care.

Stephanie and I turned up at the beginning of the outpatient clinic on a Tuesday morning to greet Mr Fraser behind an empty desk. This was my first clue. No case notes! That means your 'notes are with someone else. They weren't being typed up by his secretary. That would have been done within days of the op. Nope. Someone else has them for a bloody good reason. Stephanie either didn't see the significance or was simply not pointing it out for my benefit. The second clue was his sombre expression.

"As you may have already guessed, the news isn't good. And I hate giving bad news to good people."

I had already guessed and I'm no Sherlock. In true scientific mode, I wanted location, muscle status, prognosis, the whole Bruce Willis. Then the bomb shell. It was a T3, muscle invasive, chemotherapy as soon as the team could arrange, then at some point in the distant future, bladder removal and exploratory surgery to see if the cancer has spread.

Stephanie sat stunned as if the world had stopped turning on its axis.

I was pragmatic to a fault (and possibly maintaining my denial). I have never, not once, in life asked "why me?" Sometimes life is hard and you have to put on your crash helmet and crack on.

I asked all the usual questions of prognosis in a totally pragmatic manner. Would I need much chemotherapy? Definitely. Would I be very ill? Probably. Was it major surgery? Huge. Did I do something to bring this about? Absolutely not.

"Ok, how soon can we crack on?"

"You'll meet the Consultant Oncologist next week; she'll explain what's involved."

When we got back to the car I apologised to Stephanie for bringing this to our door. Somehow I'd done something or not done something that meant we were both in the shit for quite some time to come. We'd been married for 15 years with a couple of hospital stays between us; hers mostly by giving birth to Ari and Jonny. Mine were by doing silly stuff and breaking bits of my body but nothing on this scale.

Outside after the appointment, we sat in the car and held each other for a long time. I could feel her tears running down my neck and her sobs shaking the car's suspension. I stroked her hair in silence and watched the light rain run down the windscreen. These were surrogate tears.

I felt as though I had let her down in a spectacular way. Even if I had no way of preventing this, I was broken in a big way and was causing her huge distress. My overwhelming emotion at this point was guilt. Was I about to become a total burden? Would I need real care? Would I lose my independence or dignity? Just how ill would I become?

Baldness, sickness, diarrhoea and weight loss are most people's initial worries when cancer and chemotherapy are in their imminent future. It certainly was my fear. Stephanie and I did the "in sickness and in health" vows 15 years previously but no one really expects the sickness part to be more than a hangover, an occasional bug or a bit of man flu.

15 years objectively seems like a long time; decade and a half, one hundred and eighty months, five thousand five hundred days or so. The realisation that you might have a fraction of time left, compared to what you've had up till now, was a hellish thought. In reality the decade and a half had flown by in a flurry of activity, living and loving each other like no two people you've ever met. No two others connected or laughed or liked the same music and comedy as we did.

Stephanie and I had met in 1993. She was an Audiology student based in Glasgow Royal; the post I had vacated earlier that same year to start working in Gartnavel Hospital. My friend Donald and I were newly qualified and had been asked by Dr Slimming in Stow College to lecture on Audiology procedures for the new intake. He and I were up for anything and Dr Slimming was so thoroughly nice you could never say no to him.

On the fateful day the class turned up and Donald and I split the group in two. In my group was a stunner. She was petite at 5'2", waist length long blonde hair, black Metallica T-shirt and skin tight "painted on" denims. She was every guy's type. If you've seen the bit in Wayne's World where Garth spots his "Foxy Lady" to the Jimi Hendrix tune, then you'll know where my head was.

I volunteered her for all my practical demonstrations and refused to swap groups with Donald at the half way point. When would I ever get near a goddess like this again? Take it for what it is. She was in a different league from you, so paw her while you can. That was the last I'd be seeing her then.

"And I'll probably never see you again; yes I'll probably never see you again." (Hand in Glove by The Smiths)

The Cathouse in Glasgow is a dark and dingy rock club and some weeks later, I was there with friends when the goddess appeared wearing a black baby doll dress, fishnets and Doc Martens. It was a second Garth moment. Stephanie had apparently not minded being drooled over in front of an audience and it seems I wasn't quite as incoherent in front of beauty as I'd thought.

It was a great night and better still she agreed to another. Then another and another etc. How had I managed to bag this lady? She really was in a different league to me and still is. Her hobby for the last 11 years is Arabic Dancing. Who else, after 15 years, gets to be married to a perfect size eight belly dancer?

"She smells like angels oughta smell: the Goddess." (Marv talking about his beloved Goldie in the movie, Sin City.)

Recently, in a rare moment of rare humility, I asked what the bloody hell she saw in me. She used a car analogy to explain it. I like cars and car analogies. When Stephanie looks at me she sees a classic car. Unconventional looking (no kidding), different to the norm, rare, special and even though it requires TLC and investment to keep going, it's worthwhile having around. I like this a lot. It feeds my ego and my love of all things automotive.

We are also fortunate to have what other people regard as the best kids on the planet. Both Stephanie and I are in total agreement but it is less fluke and good fortune than it is routine and hard work. We are a tight, respectful and fun loving family group. Was I now about to break all these people's hearts? I couldn't let my goddess down. I couldn't let my kids down.

Ari is going to grow up to be a stunner just like her mum and I've got to be there to intimidate any would-be boyfriends. Jon is already a charming and funny wee man and he's just turned 9. I couldn't afford to miss a minute of these two growing up. They need their Dad. Getting through this is the only option.

"Nothing else matters" (That's a Metallica song).

I used a peculiar psychological trick to stop myself dwelling on the why and how this had come about. What in life could be worse than having cancer? If your child had cancer, that would be much, much worse. Is there any parent who wouldn't wish to exchange places with their very sick child? No probably not.

How many doting and loving parents have sat, agonising by their child's bed and wished that they could take all the pain and suffering away? I'm willing to bet every parent in a paediatric ward would give everything and more to ensure the safety of their loved one.

It wasn't until 1954 that children were allowed daily visits from parents. Until then sick kids were often placed in adult wards and had one hour on a Saturday and Sunday to see their family. That would seem inconceivable and draconian today. Sir James Spence and Sir Alan Moncrieff, both paediatricians, described how this kind of separation was traumatic to children. Their point was valid and gradual introduction of daily hospital visits were introduced.

For my part I pretended that I had been given a choice. Either of my two kids could fall ill with a life threatening condition under my watch or I could endure a trial in their stead. That would be an easy choice. I would rather take anything than sit by a bed and watch Arianne or Jonathan battle for their lives. So let's just pretend that something or someone had given me the option of taking the sickness in place of either of the kids.

It may be foolish and contrived but if there was something worse than cancer, it would be a sick and helpless child. At various stages along the journey I used the "What could be worse than this? A sick child, that's what." Pretending you had chosen an illness over their wellbeing made the worry less acute.

Breaking News

Telling friends and family is an onerous task. Not because your bringing devastating news (well partly because your dropping the C bomb on your nearest and dearest) but because of repetition. It's the same script time, after time, after time. The same worry, denial, disbelief and questions repeated on a loop. It dulls the senses upon each retelling and lessens the weight of the news to the point you're beginning to joke when you perhaps shouldn't and you become less able to see the horror on people's faces.

Early on in the diagnosis Stephanie and I had invited the family over for dinner to break the news in a single session. We both felt that dragging it out would be harder and in telling one person you were doing a disservice to the others. Mum, Dad, my brother Simon and his wife Lorraine were fully sated and sat around the table.

Once we had the dirty dishes tidied up I slipped my Oncology contact card onto the table. This is a business card with contact info of your "team." It has my oncology nurse details (Fiona) the Beatson ward number and out of hours phone details just in case you need advice.

Anne picked it up, read it and said "Whose is this?"

"It's mine, Mum."

"Someone you know?"

"No Mum, it's mine. These are people I need numbers for. I have cancer."

Silence for a heart-beat then the questions began. Anne was a nurse and a midwife for her career and understood all things medical. What followed was a full evening's dissection of all the finer details of diagnosis and treatment options. Stephanie had all of the salient facts memorised and fielded the majority of questions, for which I was grateful.

After the initial shock had worn off and once we had consensus that it would be all fine in time, the humour started. Black humour; blacker than a witch's hat. Simon is an ambulance technician and has a gory story for all occasions. We went for it, big time.

Stephanie and I have a love of black humour. Just check our Blackadder knowledge. I love Bill Hicks, George Carlin, Jimmy Carr and most comedians who push the limits. In a war footing, all jokes become black. This was definitely our war. We were preparing for the battle of our lives as a family.

Black humour is what Stephanie, Simon and I began to use. Black humour gives voice to your worst fears and ridicules them. We three did it in spades. Not everyone appreciates black humour. My Mum, as an example, was "very upset" with the three of us. That's the equivalent of saying the surface of the sun is too warm to touch. She couldn't appreciate the jokes between Simon and I.

"I get your PS3 when you die." Or "Oh well, you've had a good innings. See ya!"

Jokes about death, disfigurement, jokes about peeing into a catheter bag and a pickpocket trying to steal it. We were poking fun at a horrific situation to lessen the fear. We were actually horrifying Mum with our immaturity and upsetting her hugely in the process.

I learned that there is a time and a place for everything. Even if you personally need to vent and ridicule and blow off steam, others need sobriety and time to mull things over.

The kids were an easier pairing to break the news to, due to previous experience. Jonny's school pal, Ewan has had his left leg amputated below the knee after contracting "Ewing's sarcoma". Two years ago a lump had appeared on Ewan's shin bone and after many investigations his parents, Alison and Bobby had the bombshell dropped on them that their son had a rare form of bone cancer.

He's the exact same age as Jonny and both Stephanie and I used to balk at the idea and worry about the possibility of our kids ever getting seriously ill. How Alison and Bobby were able to function and still continue as a family unit with Ewan's Sister Olivia, remains a mystery.

At the point Ewan was about to start his chemo we tried to explain to Ari and Jonny that when we put weed killer over our whole garden it's similar in many ways to chemotherapy. The nasty weeds that were sticking out of the soil in a garden can easily be cut out (analogy to the surgery on the lump on Ewan's left leg) but what about the weeds that are too small to see? You have to treat the whole garden with chemicals to kill off the stuff below the surface.

The same is true with chemo; the chemicals kill off the body's "weeds below the surface" allowing the surgeon to cut out the lump they can see. This allowed them accessible understanding so when it came to Dad's cancer; it was simply in a different place to Ewan's, hidden from view and only visible by scans but the process would be similar.

Ewan continues to grow and thrive. He has adapted to the situation with fantastic support. He has great professionals in the back ground and a loving family in the fore ground (he even named his prosthetic leg Marcus).

Breaking the news at work was an odd process. I had lots of love from the unlikeliest of places. I have my best mate Dawn (suitably upset for me and stoic all at the same time). She has been at the Royal Infirmary since her earliest student days and we work together like a well-oiled machine. Dawn is another huge knowledge seeking Brainiac. Gym obsessed and studying obsessed; she works full time, works out all-the-damn-time and is half way through a Master's degree.

When I told her the news and likely treatment plan she was pragmatic to a fault. "No, no, you're not leaving me here on my own!", "Just get on with it and get back here." This was masking genuine affection and worry. I wasn't fooled for a second. I would definitely get on with it and be back ASAP but only partly for Dawn's benefit.

When I broke the news she temporarily stunned but quickly formed the backbone of my coping strategy at work. Dawn, like Stephanie was determined to research bladder cancer and face up to what was coming our way. She must have devoted hours and hours of her evenings looking up statistics, delving into treatment regimens, just looking for any crumb of good news to bring to work. The conversations were always aimed at being positive. Dawn was trying to keep me (and her I imagine) from sitting under a cloud of negativity.

When word spread that it was bad and I'd likely be ill for quite a while, I was getting regular, earnest one on one chats with my Senior Consultants, hugs from the junior Doctors and love from all our nursing staff. It was lovely but surreal. When you're working away, head down, you don't feel you're on most people's radar until something stunning happens. The wealth of affection was surprising as was the religious fervour.

I'm at heart, a scientist. I love evidence based science, where if a model doesn't work, the folk with big brains throw out the previous theory and start again. Who doesn't love Professor Hawking, Marie Curie, Pasteur, Einstein, Galileo, Dawkins and Hitchens? As for the latter, lots of people have no love for Christopher Hitchens. At some point I have read all his books and I've loved his work since I first read "God is not Great".

In his final book of essays "Mortality" Hitchens charted his thought processes on finding out he had terminal oesophageal cancer. He charted his final days in a literary euphemism by travelling from Wellsville to Tumour Town. Unshakeable in his absence of faith, it was seminal prose from a truly enlightened man.

My recurring memory from the book is the phrase "I am sixty -one. In whatever kind of race "life" may be, I have very abruptly become a finalist". He died on 15th December 2011

Naturally, lots of his work is contentious and opinionated. It's designed to provoke a reaction from theists. The fact remains as an atheist I was touched by the number of people who were regularly "praying for me". People who I would have never, not ever, have thought religious were thinking of me and praying I'd do well. It was a genuine pleasant surprise to be so well regarded.

I still though was banking my beliefs on scientific medicine and a skilled surgeon (or a few as it turned out).

Manchester

Stephanie and I had an eagle eye view over the stage at the Manchester Evening News arena. We were having a weekend away for Stephanie's birthday and we had travelled three hours south on the M6 to see Radiohead play live. Our kids were being baby sat by my parents and we had booked a hotel for a couple of days, just to make it all the more memorable.

This was a pre-treatment, last gasp treat for the two of us. Neither of us could predict when I would next be able to enjoy a holiday. So we decided to go the whole hog. A break in a city we had never been to, a band we both loved, sightseeing, meals out and alcohol.

We abandoned the car at the hotel and used the tram to get around. Manchester's trams were the best integrated transport system either of us had ever seen. It enabled us to hop on and off to see the Manchester sights.

Hours and hours were spent wandering around in unseasonably warm autumnal weather. The trams allowed us to flit from one side of the city to the other in no time. It was a café culture equal to any modern European city. We spent a thoroughly enjoyable afternoon in the Lowry museum and the National War museum.

We came across a beautiful water fountain lit up with multi coloured lights. Jets of water shot out of the ground in a rhythmic display, all changing tempo and hue every few seconds. I took some choice pictures of Stephanie in the middle of the water. A stop mid-afternoon saw us topping up on our caffeine reserves. Dinner was in Chinatown at the most authentic Chinese restaurant I've ever seen. Then off to the arena to see the band.

Our seats were in a private box, high up in the gods. The stage was off to our right and the view was incredible. The arena lay below us, vast and crowded. Stephanie and I were riding on a high after a cracking day. I even brazenly approached Pete Turner, bassist from the band Elbow, to thank him personally for the contribution to my music library. He seemed a little shocked at being accosted but he was very polite all the same.

The band was visually and audibly stunning, we've seen them live lots of times. Massive screens showed close-ups of each member interspersed with impressionist colours. It was an immersive experience, delivered by consummate professionals. Radiohead never fail to impress.

Then it happened. "How to disappear completely" started. A favourite song of mine but I had never given much thought to its lyrics. It's ethereal, mostly instrumental with only fifteen lines of lyrics and builds very slowly to an orchestral crescendo, all the while Thom Yorke sings:

In a little while I'll be gone.

The moment's already past.

Yeah it's gone.

I'm not here. This isn't happening.

I'm not here. I'm not here.

I suddenly had a huge lump in my throat. Tears were building up in my eyes. What the hell was going on? What's this? A realisation had taken right until this point to catch up with me.

I have cancer.

"We know that", said another atavistic part of my brain. "This news is old. Get over yourself. Don't be such a giant wimp."

But, I have cancer!

"Yeah? So? Are you looking for a medal or something? You're not the only one. Lots of people are in worse situations. Grow up."

The fact had hit home like a thunderclap. "I have cancer." It was now a vast mountain looming over me. The shadow it cast for that brief instant felt overwhelming. This was an impossible climb. It was a peak of foreboding deadly indifference.

The song had lifted a mirror to my denial. I'm not here. This isn't happening. I'm not here. The music lasted nearly six minutes; a cathartic six minutes of indulgent surrender to fear and worry.

Stephanie let me deal with it and I excused myself and went to the gents. Some cold water and a brief break was all that was needed. There was no running away from it. It was here and couldn't be ignored. I gathered myself and the rest of the gig and the weekend for that matter, were outstanding. My rude awakening to the larger picture was a blip, that's all.

If it were a metaphorical mountain to be climbed then it was best to concentrate on each step at a time. Looking up at the whole thing simply made me dizzy with perspective.

The other, less sympathetic part of my brain whispered to itself:

"You're such a big girl's blouse."

Chemo

Jan Wallace (Consultant Oncologist) explained how three cycles of chemotherapy, or four if your body could cope, would take me to the New Year and shrink the tumour sufficiently for the surgical team to successfully remove it all.

She had squeezed Stephanie and I in at the end of a hellish busy clinic as a favour to Mr Fraser, skipping lunch in the process. This was in order to get the ball rolling on my treatment.

My chemo regime would be week 1; big dose. Week 2 would be a smaller dose of a specific chemical. Week 3 would be a week off to recover. Then repeat in multiples till the scans showed sufficient improvement for surgery to begin.

Ms Wallace is based at The Beatson Oncology centre; attached to Gartnavel General Hospital in Glasgow's west end. The centre is named after Dr George Beatson, later Sir George Beatson, who was appointed surgeon to the 1890s Glasgow Cancer and Skin Institution.

The new Beatson is plush modern and completely terrifying (mainly because if you're there, you are in deep trouble). It has an ultra-modern high atrium, full glass frontage, free Wi-Fi access, a plush café and scores of bald people holding onto drip stands, chain smoking at the entrance.

The irony wasn't lost on me and the amount of cigarette butts on the ground was utterly depressing.

"O would some power the giftie gie us to see ourselves as others see us." (Robert Burns: To a Louse)

In 1954 Sir Richard Doll and Sir Austin Bradford Hill published a study in the British Medical Journal. It was a study of lung cancer patients undertaken in twenty London hospitals. Rather than the expected culprits, coal fires, motor exhaust or tar macadam, there was the first clear correlation between lung cancer and smoking.

"It (lung cancer) may be fifty times as great among those who smoke twenty five cigarettes a day as among non-smokers."

An unofficial online biography states that the cancer link to cigarettes spurred Sir Richard to immediately quit smoking and he died of an unrelated illness in 2005, aged 92. I would like to think that it's true, even though I couldn't find any corroborating reports.

Chemo week one began with my first big dose. This was an eleven hour overnighter in one of the Beatson wards. Nine different chemicals were changed back to back from early evening through till dark o'clock in the morning. I was attached to a drip, stuck in bed with the "Alaris" pump beeping every hour and a half to signal the nurse to hang the next bag of goodies.

The Alaris is a small, blue coloured machine with dozens of buttons and lights which attaches half way up a standard drip stand. It measures and delivers accurate dosages from a bag suspended above, droning, groaning, beeping and pulsing as it pumps your prescribed poison.

Sleep was optional. Not least due to the fact that four and a half litres of chemicals need to go somewhere. Having to pee into bottles half hourly was a drag. Having to do it with an audience of three other blokes in a four bedded room was worse. Using a toilet wasn't going to happen. The wheelchair was no use to me as one arm was occupied with a drip in it. I effectively had one remaining useful limb.

My initial coyness and trying desperately to hide my ministrations under a hospital sheet, quickly gave way to a "to hell with this" attitude as I was peeing so often. So knob out, peeing into a bottle, regardless of who was present became the norm. Dignity? Please check yours in at the door; you will not be requiring it for the foreseeable future.

A week later it was time for the smaller dose. This was done as an outpatient, usually on a Tuesday afternoon, for a couple of hours. This dosage was a minor top up of the specific bladder tumour targeted chemo. This was not nearly as long as the big dose and by far more sociable.

The outpatient room was outfitted with large, plush dental looking chairs. Perhaps as many as 10 chairs around the periphery of the room each with a client hooked to an Alaris, reading, some sleeping, many munching the free sandwiches and tea and biscuits.

It was on my first of outpatient session and thinking back to all my previous clinic visits that I realised, I'd seen no one my age. Not by half. Not even close. It was an unending sea of grey. I was the odd man out.

If this is indicative of ever increasing cancer rates, then Ms Wallace is going to miss even more lunch breaks in the future than she currently does. The NHS has an elephant in the room which is growing larger and larger by the year: an aging population.

The better my NHS becomes at keeping people fit and healthy, the greater the strain on resources. Cancers are statistically far more common the older you become. By 2011 the number of people 65 years and over was 10.4 million. That's set to rise to 15.8 million by the time we reach 2030. That's only 17 years away.

An increasingly aging patient group need ever more resources, not less. Yet the NHS needs to find £15-20 billion in savings in the next two years and still attempt to maintain care at the current levels.

"I hope I die before I get old." (My Generation by The Who). No one listens to The Who much nowadays.

Week three was my week off. This was a misnomer by a large factor. The week off is where all the chemicals conspire to show you their real side effects. The potential list of side effects is huge and not everyone gets them all. You do get a handy red book to document your particular set, not that any health care professional ever looked at mine.

I assumed it was for self-gratification to see if you'd collected the full set (just like Panini football stickers). My main effects came from the Cisplatin in my cocktail of drugs. These were tiredness, tinnitus, massive hyperacusis and hearing loss.

The tiredness wasn't just a lethargic kind of weariness. No, this was a bone deep, cellular absence of energy that had to be experienced to be believed. I have gone to the gym three times per week since I was sixteen, usually before work starts. I can lift massive weights, only upper body of course, much more than the vast majority of others. You can gird yourself at the gym and overcome simple tiredness. Regular gorillas at the gym will shout at one another "dig deep!", "push it!", "max the envelope!" and all the other motivational bullshit to fulfil their sets. This was just not possible on chemo. When you ran down there was no lower you could dig.

The Cisplatin also damages the hair cells within the ear's cochlea. The high frequency hair cells are most often affected and this gives the world a bass heavy sound. I love rock music;

often with the bass turned up but this is hopeless for speech. Lots of meaning bearing consonants are in the high frequency region and once they are lost sentences take on weird meanings.

"A dreadful smell of leather" and "A dreadful spell of weather" are dependent on just a few high frequency sounds. During one consultation I once thought a doctor told me "Your testicles are black." Before I embarrassed myself, my IQ kicked in and I realised he'd said "Your test results are back."

Alarmingly, I could barely follow anyone's speech but if someone put down a fork, closed a door or farted marginally too loud, I'd collapse in a noise induced heap. Common sounds were coming across with the force of an atomic explosion. This is sensitivity within the cochlea due to absorption of the chemo making the supposedly desensitised hair cells react suddenly once the received stimulus breaks through.

Fortunately this is my area of expertise and I knew these were likely to be temporary side effects and would stop once the chemo was over. This was still long months away though.

The Acoustic Properties of Hospital Curtains

Early in the Chemo stages I was exposed to another's "End of Life" conversation. This would have a profound effect on my view of my own treatment. I just wasn't aware of the significance until much later. It was late in the evening and I was in Beatson ward 6 for my first overnight chemo session. Another young bloke and I were the only two occupants in a four bedded room.

This guy had to be in his late teens or early twenties; it was hard to be sure. He was completely bald, ashen grey to the point of being transparent and swollen from all the chemicals.

He was attached to his own Alaris, sitting in a chair. He was awkwardly positioned, obviously pained but stoically bearing it with good humour. Two visitors were with him; his girl-friend and his brother. It was unmistakably his brother. The similarities were obvious as were the contrasts.

His brother was as healthy and vibrant as he was pale and wan. These blokes were possibly twins, being so similar in age. However put both face to face across a sheet of glass and they could have been a modern manifestation of Dorian Gray.

His consultant came to have a word and asked if he wished to have his visitors present for the consultation. The doctor had brought a chair and pulled the curtain around this guy's bed and his family. His name was Steven. A short summary was issued on what he had endured thus far which I felt was incredible. His treatments had been varied and torturous. Surgery, chemo and radiotherapy had all been administered in multiples judging by the conversation.

The doctor laid out the treatment options available from here on in. "Limited" was the word most often repeated in the conversation. It was now simple mathematics. Steven's body was overcome by fast replicating cells in multiple organs and nothing could stop the irreversible tide. With each treatment regime Steven's body became weaker and his cancer remained unabated. His battle was being lost faster than it could be fought. Medicine had no more ammunition to try and time was now short.

Steven may well have been prepared for the inevitable news but his brother and girlfriend definitely were not. Angry accusations were aimed at the consultant and anguish and recriminations from both visitors could be heard far and wide. As far as they were concerned there must have been some avenue left unexplored. Some up and coming cancer drug had yet to be tried and Steven needed it now. The doctor couldn't have been better or more patient.

He had all the time in the world for these people and his explanations were accurate without being too technical, considerate without being patronising and above all professionally empathetic. He was extremely well versed in this sort of counselling, which was depressing in and of itself. He must have delivered this same news many, many times.

Steven was equally capable in what must have been the lowest point in a very short and hard life. He thanked his consultant for his patience and expertise. He explained that his girlfriend and brother would be ok once he'd had a chance to reiterate that all had been done that could have, in his exhaustive journey.

I hated being privy to this. I was pinned to an Alaris machine and unable to leave. These people needed the kind of privacy that an insubstantial hospital curtain couldn't provide. It was horribly intrusive. The defining moment of three people's lives was happening six feet away and I was an interloper. I was utterly ashamed because I felt like the worst kind of gate crasher.

I began to get upset for all three of them. I was beginning to get choked up on their behalf. Oh shit, this can't happen! I was not allowed to wallow in others' grief. I was starting to flush with embarrassment. I took out the phone and a pair of headphones from my bag and stuck the mp3 player on as loud as I could tolerate.

I now couldn't hear the rest of the conversation but despite the blaring music I couldn't help but dwell on mortality. Would I get one of these "talks" at some point in the future? Possibly. Would I be as calm and capable as Steven had been? Probably not but I hoped so.

He had been the strong one of the three. Steven had strength of personality greater than his years. He was helping them to understand that the doctors, nurses and numerous unseen health service workers had done everything possible. Yet this was still not enough for him to survive cancer.

He and I shared a few pleasantries over the course of a single day and he seemed ordinary in every way. He was extraordinary in the calm acceptance and almost serene support he was providing for his loved ones. Here were two people who would soon be going on with their lives without him.

If I were to leave Stephanie, Arianne and Jonathan I hoped beyond hope I could be as brave and stoic as that bloke. They sat together well into the night, all three of them. Steven was supporting them both in the most admirable and pragmatic way.

He was the rock on which they broke their hearts that night. Later a song came on by Pearl Jam and ever since that night I think of Steven:

"And where ever you've gone and wherever we might go
It don't seem fair. You seemed to like it here.
Your light reflected now, reflected from afar.
We were but stones. Your light made us stars."
(Light Years by Pearl Jam)

Bottle Crashing

After the first cycle of chemotherapy, I'd begged to get back to work. I thought, in my arrogance, I was coping just fine and there was no reason I couldn't do some good back at Royal Infirmary HQ. I was prepared to take holiday leave on my treatment days and get back to feeling useful and worthwhile the rest of the working week. Occupational Health agreed I could work in administration but with a strict rule of no patient contact.

Their reasoning was I was immuno-suppressed and at risk from the public. The head of O.H., Rona (preferential professional treatment again) was not to be trifled with and discretion is the better part of valour. I decided I would do anything and everything Rona said to get back to work. Stephanie was justifiably sceptical (worried I would overdo things and make matters worse) but for the sake of my sanity she didn't resist.

My line manager, Forbes was totally supportive. He would be forced to cover the majority of my clinical hours. Forbes was a manager for many years and now he'd be doing two jobs. One as administrator for all of Audiology in Greater Glasgow and Clyde and one as a clinician trying to see my list of patients for me.

It was a thankless task for the man but he agreed that there was still a place for me in clinic, in whatever capacity I could manage. This meant a massive restriction of duties for me and an equal escalation for him.

So, working on a Monday, Tuesday and Wednesday, I would then admit myself to ward 6 in the Beatson at 5pm on the Wednesday evening for the overnighter. Annual leave would give me the Thursday and Friday to recover, plus the weekend.

I went back to work on the Monday, then Tuesday as the top up afternoon and normal working the rest of the week. It was during cycle two's top up that my "bottle crashed" in a big way.

Like everyone on the planet, life throws stressors at you at various points along the way and you find a way to get by. It's perfectly normal when some people throw a bit of a fit or an emotional outburst through stress. Some folk have a tendency not to cope with seemingly mild stress factors; a select few however need instructing on methods of coping.

Quite a few I've seen professionally for Tinnitus counselling. These sufferers require careful coaching and often need to be shown the skills. I'd like to think that up till now I could win an award as most "calm in the face of adversity".

Not prone to outbursts, no crying at how unfair it all is, no temper to speak of, nor shying away from difficulties, I try to be level headed and problem solving as opposed to "freaky mental". I have never had a panic attack, for instance.

However, cycle two top up was half an hour old when I happened to put my book down for a minute and looked round the room at the other people in their glorified dental chairs. It was that age gap again that bothered me. I was half the age of most others here.

Their cancer was surely a factor of free radical's build up versus time, or more likely, a lifestyle choice making cancer if not inevitable then highly bloody likely. I was becoming irrational and didn't see what was coming.

How many in this room smoked like a chimney? Or drank like an alcoholic? What had you done, old man, to warrant being here? What about you, old lady? What nasty habits have you kept up to warrant being here? I've done none of that. Christopher Hitchens had another memorable phrase that never leaves me:

"To the dumb question "Why me?" the cosmos barely bothers to return the reply: "Why not?""

A sudden cold sweat hit me like a shower. A broken glass sensation went off in my brain.

"There's been a mistake."

"I'm not supposed to be here."

"I'm not one of you lot. I'm way too young for this shit."

"I have to go, really! I've got to leave. NOW!"

The dialogue was all in my head but it was overpowering. I couldn't possibly stay; the urge to leave was just too strong. I started looking at my Alaris machine in a blind panic to see how to power it off.

It was just a sea of buttons and lights. I had seen it done before by others but for love nor money I couldn't remember how to do it. I could just yank the needle from my arm and do a runner. Leave! Oh fuck, please let me leave! Please?

The cascade of breaking glass was getting worse. I was losing it. I was starting to shake. Someone's going to see then they'll never let me out. Stop trembling! Someone's going to see! Stop shaking! Stop! Where is the power button? Just pull the needle out of the vein and let's go! Pull it out, now!

My peripheral vision was going and I was in full blown panic mode. No rational thoughts, I was gasping like a fish out of water and my sight was blurry. Any second now I was going to pass out. I was on a downward spiral. I could see only pin pricks of light and was aware of my chest heaving up and down. My heart was about to burst. Fuck, I'm dying.

Wait and breathe. Just wait a second, breathe. That's it Paul. One more second and another breath will do. Let's go for another breath, and another. Well done.

The fog gradually lifted and a welcome wave of calm came from the top of my head and passed all the way down through me. It had passed as quick as it had come. No more than a couple of minutes had passed beginning to end according to the clock on the wall. More importantly no one had noticed. I had managed to meltdown totally and recover without a single person seeing it happen.

I spent the next hour or so going over my "meltdown" in detail and the sensations I was left with. I laughed at the absurdity of what had happened inside minutes. I was grinning like a moron. Not so cool and scientific now are you? You're a bottle crashing wanker just like everyone else!

In arrogantly priding myself on being unflappable, my ego had taken a sound kick in the nuts and I was all the better for it. The King James Bible contains the original longer version of the saying but the shorter version was just as apt; "Pride cometh before the fall."

The sociability of the Top Up Tuesdays (coining a phrase) was mostly head nodding and acknowledging one another's presence or asking polite "how many treatments have you got left?" type of thing. Most, if not all, brought their own entertainment.

The number of silver surfers I came across with iPads eBook readers and netbooks was staggering. Judging by this lot, the nation's pensions were all being spent in PC World. There was one guy though, who sorely needed some other form of entertainment, who tortured me for a whole Tuesday afternoon.

I had just been hooked up to my Alaris when a voice next to me said;

"This place is utter crap!"

This turned out to be the kind of guy who is never happy. Not ever. Not with anything or anyone. "Jim" had a hearing aid that he bought (at considerable expense) from a dispenser on the high street as apparently the NHS ones were "Utter crap."

I was willing to give him the benefit of the doubt, he may well be having a bad day or a low mood but as the session wore on my sympathies died along with my good humour.

The hearing aid dispenser apparently was "A highway robber" and seems to have ripped him off with a second rate device. I was then regaled by his many visits to his long suffering Optician, whose specs are "Utter crap". His Podiatrist's shoe inserts are (can you guess), "Utter crap". His home help apparently doesn't. He is widowed (he seems to think she did it was out of spite) and his sons never visit: I can't imagine why.

If the Playboy mansion sent a bus full of naked bunnies round to "Jim's" house to personally deliver his lottery cheque, he'd complain that the champagne was too warm.

His most endearing trait, by far, was to have had every conceivable disease, condition, malady and injury worse than anyone in the history of mankind. From a broken this, to a dose of that, "Jim" had it first, for longer and much worse than you or I.

"Cancer?"

"Uh, yeah mate, I've got cancer."

"Not like mine, you don't."

What followed was a blow by blow account of "Jim's" liver cancer. It was a comprehensive study of his medical maladies. From the agony of his partial liver removal all the way through to his disastrous diarrhoea on chemo cycle one (including a part where his home help had to peel him from his undershorts),

"Jim" was determined to make me grateful for being so lucky in the cancer stakes. All nurses were "Idiots", all doctors were "Butchers" and the Beatson clinic was a "Waiting room for the nearly dead."

All my defence of the NHS and its huge commitment to the welfare of the UK was derided and sneered at. No way was I about to divulge that I was part of the establishment. I would have simply painted a target on my forehead for his wrath. This comedian was a self-absorbed, self-pitying, dour bastard and for the second session in a row I wanted to rip the needle from my arm and bolt.

Two and a half hours equals 150 minutes and "Jim" made me feel as if each and every one was dragging by. The sketch in "Airplane" where Ted recounts his and Elaine's doomed love to other passengers, totally unaware that they're committing suicide beside him: that was "Jim" and I.

Nodding sagely at appropriate points, I'd idly wonder if jabbing a biro in my eye or sucking farts from a dead seagull could be less painful than this. 150 minutes passed at "the pace of an asthmatic ant, carrying some heavy shopping" (Blackadder quote again) and at long last, I was free.

My machine had beeped its final chorus and I was already wrapping up the one sided conversation with platitudes to "Jim" whilst trying to catch a nurse's eye. I was off as quick as humanly possible with polite wishes that he would feel better soon and it wasn't long now etc. One of the nurses unhooked me from my machine and showed me to the door with a parting, "Looks like you made a friend there."

"Lucky me." Was all I could muster whilst belting down the corridor (away from him) as fast as my wheels could go.

(Over)Doing it?

The latter part of the year saw a routine of sorts at work. Forbes was "front of the house" working in clinic with Dawn. I was office bound and feeling weird. Three differences were in evidence that made each day seem like the Twilight Zone.

No client contact. I'd been a clinician for twenty plus years and now being tied to a desk was terrible. Working with clients was the best part of the job. There is nothing that compares to "switching on" a pair of modern hearing aids and watching the varied reactions people have. It's hilarious and entertaining and rewarding all at once. Admin gives none of the "job well done" gratification, even if you've put your heart and soul into it.

No uniform. I was going to work in civvies for the first time in an age. Without a uniform (ours is Ocean Blue top and dark blue combats) you don't feel like a team player. I was deliberately instructed not to wear scrubs as I was forbidden to see clients without them. This was a dis-incentive for me specifically.

The rest of our clinic knew I would be inclined just to "pitch in" if things got busy and wore my uniform. In denims and a t-shirt I look like a patient. If you saw a disabled bloke in a clinic the presumption would be, he's waiting to be taken for his appointment. Not, there goes the boss of the department.

Thirdly, was the overpowering nausea. The Beatson clinic issued a cornucopia of chemicals to combat sickness. As explained to me, it's essential not to start being sick as it becomes harder to stop. Once vomiting begins, the medicine becomes harder to keep down, therefore it's less effective and therefore you're more likely to vomit, and so on.

The anti-emetic meds are strictly four hourly; very strictly four hourly. Even at night you are encouraged to take them at the prescribed interval. Only by keeping on top of the sickness can you reasonably expect to keep food, strength and medicines intact.

Lots of people have come unstuck during treatment by failing to keep control on the meds, then being sick and falling into a downward spiral. Ultimately if you can't limit the sickness you then need admission into hospital for IV anti-emetics. I'd go all-out to avoid that nonsense.

I had all sorts of reminders. I had bleeps on my Samsung. Microsoft Outlook reminders were set on the PC. My watch had an alarm (which I suddenly couldn't hear due to the chemo). I never forgot to take my sickness tabs. It was all the more galling then to still feel sick to my stomach all day, every day.

Regular food and little portion sizes were the order of the day but everything took effort to keep down. Distractions helped to keep your mind off the nausea but not always. Forbes walked into my office one time to find me hunched over my bin, willing myself not to be sick into it.

My loved ones started a new mantra. "Are you sure you're not overdoing it?" During the day it was a Dawn chorus. "You OK? Sure you're up to this?" I know it was concern and affection but she watched me like a hawk every day, looking for signs that I was fading. I was trying to hide the signs as best as I could.

Stephanie's concern was compounded by the rest of the family. They would ask her the same "Are you sure he's not overdoing it?" but in part it was an accusation. She had personal concern double that of anyone else. She also had guilt laden from others that perhaps she should somehow be able to put a stop to all this. I definitely wasn't helping.

A casual discussion could escalate in to a disagreement, ultimately to an argument. I was expending what little energies I had at work so that by home time I was a spent bag of bones. She rightly felt aggrieved that work was getting the best of me, leaving her and the kids with less. Quality and quantity family time was now slim pickings.

"How are you feeling?"

"Fine."

"You sure?"

"Yep."

"Are you sure you're not overdoing it?"

"Nah. Piece of piss."

"You're looking really tired. Maybe you'd want a lie down for an hour?"

"Nope. I'm OK."

I could so easily have given in, crawled under a quilt and had any number of duvet days but I needed to pretend I was capable for her. Self-image and arrogance pushed me to turn up each day to work, give what I could and go home wrecked and useless for my wife. Looking back, I know now I was torturing her. It was stressing her out on a daily basis. I was selling my loved ones short in the worst way. In the pretence that I was OK, but obviously not, I cast her concerns aside.

It was the worst sort of bullshit machismo and I was pretending to myself as much as to my wife.

I was in denial as bad as Monty Python's Black Knight:

There's a short battle between King Arthur and the Black Knight at the end of which Arthur easily cuts off both the Black Knight's arms. The right arm comes off second, causing it and the black knight's sword to drop to the ground. Blood comically jets freely from the stump.

Arthur: Victory is mine!

He is kicked onto his backside by the black knight.

Black Knight: Come on, then! (Kicking Arthur again)

Arthur: What?

Black Knight: Have at you!

Arthur: You are indeed brave, sir knight, but the fight is mine!

Black Knight: Oohhh, had enough, eh?

Arthur: Look, **you stupid bastard**, you've got no arms left!

Black Knight: Yes I have!

Arthur: LOOK! (As he incredulously points to both arms lying on the ground)

Black Knight: 'tis but a flesh wound, my lord.

The worst fate I could have imagined at this point was to be at home, alone. That meant no company. I am very much, a social animal and need other people around and it would mean plenty of time to dwell. No thank you, I needed to keep myself occupied and distracted.

A routine that's a struggle is after all, still a routine. I didn't and couldn't see the distress I was causing Stephanie. She was watching her guy drag himself out of bed to get to work, looking pale sick and tired, all the while pretending he had nothing but "a flesh wound." I was definitely being a stupid bastard.

And I knew it.

The Hard Part is Over?

The last couple of cycles of chemo brought us up to Christmas. By this point my energy levels and tolerance to the chemicals was at an all-time low. Ms Wallace had done weekly blood tests and decided a fourth cycle was tolerable, just. My earlier arrogance of coping on cycle one had made way to utter exhaustion by cycle four. My low ebb may go some way to explaining my behaviour towards the visit I'd had from a volunteer "spiritual counsellor".

Tucked up in the hospital bed, with occasional beeps from my Alaris, my door flew open (someone tell me, why does no one knock in a hospital?) and the tiniest, most devoutly religious "wee" woman just burst in. I wasn't jumping to conclusions about her religious leanings; the most gargantuan wooden crucifix, complete with Christ's head hanging low was around her neck.

How did she manage to walk with this thing? It was huge, massive, impressively detailed all the same, but Jesus! Perhaps it was a penance or then again if Christ did carry his own cross up to Golgotha, perhaps she was issuing a challenge to "Him" by lugging this around her neck.

"Can I talk to you about our lord Jesus Christ?"

My heart sank. She was as lively as Ricky Fulton's Reverend I.M. Jolly. Our hospital chaplain in Glasgow Royal is Adam, the antithesis to this lady. He is ex RAF and the most fun, charming and friendly bloke you could meet.

Adam turned up to reception one day in our clinic, simply to introduce himself as the new chaplain and happened to ask for batteries for his hearing aid. I was appalled. He was wearing a massive NHS aid that was as outdated as it was ugly.

I asked if he was currently busy and marched him into a clinical room. An assessment and two new aids followed. Preferential treatment goes both ways and a friendship was formed at the same time.

We may not see eye to eye on the sole topic of religion but he's a real mate, having joined me for weekly chats in the department since I got ill. He probably has ulterior motives for hanging around so much. Maybe hoping I'll crack and find God. Sorry Adam, it isn't going to happen.

This lady however was monotone in the extreme and bore an expression that suggested she sucked on lemons for a hobby. I didn't have the energy to be my usual patient and smiley self. Similarly, I could hardly feign Tourette's and abuse the woman for her chosen profession.

"Sorry mate, you'd be wasting your time on me I'm afraid. I'm an atheist."

She looked at me. I smiled gently, inoffensively. She looked some more. A long time passed. An uncomfortably long period of silence followed. Had she not understood me? Had I somehow answered in Klingon by mistake? Excruciating silence ensued. My smile was waning due to muscle fatigue. It was now a battle of wills, who would be forced to speak first? Not me.

Our common ground as far as I was concerned, was nil. Plus, if I waited long enough, surely she'd pitch forward with the weight of that thing around her neck. That would be worth a few more minutes of my valuable time.

"You do realise, we're talking about your immortal soul in not accepting our lord into your life?"

Hah! You lose. I out "silenced" you. Triumph. Ok, it was a small victory but I was still gutted that she hadn't toppled over. She must have a spine of solid stone.

"Sorry, honestly, I'm very convinced by evolution and science. I'm not even remotely religious. I just don't believe in the things that you do, I'm afraid." No reply from her so I ploughed on.

"Honestly, really, there's nothing you say that could convince me that there's a god." She gave me a blank stare, and even more silence.

Still remained mute. This cannot go on. It's a war of attrition. She may never leave unless I swear an undying love for her god. The Alaris machine signalled a change of chemicals. I was never so happy to see a nurse appear.

"Sorry, you'll have to excuse us as I need to change over Paul's bag."

I could have hugged and kissed this staff nurse, even if he wasn't my type. When the volunteer had gone the nurse said:

"She's bloody hard work, that one!" I laughed. You have no idea mate.

*

As an example of what chemo does to you, one time, on a walk around Drumpellier Country Park I hit a wall worse than a marathon runner. Lap one had been fine, pushing the chair at Stephanie's walking pace whist the kids cycled round and around. It was bright but certainly not warm.

It was the kind of perfect sunny, wintry day where long walks stave off the cold and you conceivably could just keep going until hunger forced you to stop. Half way round the second time and the tank ran dry. My batteries ran completely flat. The wind went out of my sails. You get the picture by now. I couldn't move another inch.

I was gulping in the air and my head was beginning to swim. My hands felt like I was wearing boxing gloves. Each time I tried to push the chair, I couldn't feel the wheels. I looked as though I'd suddenly developed Parkinson's.

I stopped and mock cuddled my wife to prevent myself from keeling over. Stephanie kindly reciprocated but I wasn't improving in a hurry and she had to push me the rest of the way back to the car (no mean feat since the chair hasn't any push handles).

Never before had I ground to a complete halt with no means of going on. It was a big blow to the ego to be assisted like a true invalid and fears were beginning to materialise of being a burden.

Likewise, Christmas was a flurry of brief activity and sudden exhaustion. At times I had to excuse myself and simply lie down. In my parent's house with Simon and Lorraine, my wife, kids and parents in attendance a mist descended and I had the overwhelming urge to fall down on the carpet and sleep.

Instead I used their spare bed for an hour and woke fresh as a daisy. It was the suddenness that was so disconcerting, one minute you're fine, the next, zilch. Best find a place to lie down, soon.

The latter two overnight cycles of chemo were in a single room, which was a bonus. Dawn would visit straight from work. I had been working Wednesdays in Gartnavel to allow me to go straight to the Beatson.

Dawn would finish her afternoon clinic, then travel farther into the city, the opposite direction to her commute, in order to spend some time with me. She was lengthening her day and her journey to keep me company.

Stephanie then would bring the kids in later for the hour's visiting time. This broke the long evening up until about eight o'clock. Then I'd watch some TV on my Samsung phone using the free Wi-Fi and try to nap between Alaris beeps. Energy conservation was now an issue as were a lack of eyebrows. It is singularly the oddest thing to see your reflection with no eyebrows.

The hair loss thing for a bloke is no biggie (insert your own Bruce Willis gag here). I had thinned way out on top but wasn't totally bald. I'm sure the devastation for women losing their hair is a huge blow in self-esteem but for blokes it's less of an issue. My eyebrows though were non-existent.

My eyes are my most complemented factor by a long margin. Very pale blue, inherited from Anne and all the more obvious without dark eyebrows shading them. I was ashen grey and shattered all the time and puffy from all the chemicals. Almost but not quite bald and yet I was still getting compliments from nursing staff about my eyes. How super.

The final overnight stay ended around 4am and I was so ecstatic I begged the ward sister to discharge me so I could drive home and catch the last couple of hours in bed with my wife. She looked at me as if I'd just spit in her coffee.

This was not the "done thing", leaving a hospital in the middle of the night. Too bad, I'd have to wait till the shift change at eight am. Not to be dismissed, I resorted to begging. I just wanted a celebratory cuddle that it was the last cycle.

I appealed to her feminine, romantic side; simply wishing to surprise the love of my life with an impromptu gesture of affection. After much prostate begging, she relented and I shot off up Great Western Road like an inmate on parole. Instead of a welcome embrace however I just succeeded in scaring the shit out of Stephanie by appearing in the middle of the room, in the middle of the night. I promptly lay down and went into a sound sleep but she couldn't.

Ms Wallace was delighted with the final scan results. The chemotherapy had done just what we'd collectively hoped for. The cancer was reduced to a large degree, the anatomy all around seemed largely unaffected, and in short the tumour was ripe for the picking.

It was time to meet the surgeon who would be doing me the favour of a lifetime. The hard part was surely over. Recover from what was to be major surgery and life for Stephanie, the kids and I would return to normal.

Consultations

John Crooks was running through all the risky parts that could go wrong in surgery. He and his colleague Mr Rajan, were the consultants who, in a month's time would be dissecting my innermost viscera. It was early January and we were consulting in Stobhill Hospital. I was cool, calm and asked all of the most pertinent questions.

A report was published in March 1967 which was phlegmatically called: Organisation of Medical Work in Hospitals. It's better known as The Cogwheel report due to the meshed gear graphic on its front cover. This paper tried to bridge the mistrust that had developed between hospitals and doctors. It called for greater integration of doctors in the actual management of hospital affairs, prior to which was solely the job of trustees.

It also recommended (along with the Salmon report in 1967) that medicine divide itself into specialties and sub-specialties. This had a huge effect on current medical practice. From that point ever greater sub-divisions in medicine split up and concentrated in ever greater detail within a particular field. Even now, the consultants I work for super-specialise into ear, nose or throat.

Mr Crooks was a specialist in Urology. His field was one of kidneys, bladder and ureters. I would, at every available opportunity, proffer the phrase "The Waterworks Clinic."

No Stephanie this time. We both had turned a corner to do what had to be done. No more tears or histrionics, each new step would be one step closer to a cancer free future. I would attend the clinic appointments and report back what the big bosses said.

Mr Crooks was a gentleman consultant. Lots of other supposedly professional people I've met as a peer, subordinate and patient could take lessons from this man. He had a reputation for bloody good surgery and as a caring and thoughtful clinician to boot. He was kind to a fault and gave lots of time in his clinic to discuss my expectations and likely recovery time.

It turns out I needed a month to recover my physiology from the ravages of chemo, if I was to make it out the other side of surgery. Most interesting of all the information Mr Crooks had, was the possibility of "building" a new bladder, from a section of large bowel. Of all the down sides that could go wrong with the operation, the thought of not having bags hanging on the outside of my body appealed in a big way.

"Mike Palmer." Mr Crooks had now volunteered yet another consultant, Mr Palmer, to do a double act on me in what was becoming an ever more complex undertaking. Mr Crooks and Mr Rajan would remove the bladder and as much else as he could for histology to test the extent of the cancer and Mr Palmer would then take over to reconstruct a neo-bladder from a suitable section of large bowel.

It could take as long as 11 hours to finish the job. I was a one man, full working day for the surgeons and theatre staff. The cost of NHS treatment for one individual for one ailment was spiralling. I'm by no means an isolated case or by a long margin the most costly. As the hair advert says, "I'm worth it."

These guys were the perfect age for surgeons, just old enough to be extremely experienced. Not too old that coordination and eyesight were suffering. These were professionals who had been there, seen that and bought the t-shirt. Just so long as neither one was a closet alcoholic or prescribed his own pain meds, I would be in the best of hands. Reassurance and competence leaked from them like an aura.

My appointment at Mr Palmer's clinic was a few days prior to the proposed operation date at Gartnavel General. I was bang on time but he wasn't. "Mr Palmer's clinic is running forty five minutes late." called the receptionist. I was glad I always have a book with me on my phone. Five minutes later,

"Mr Palmer's clinic is now running sixty minutes late." this receptionist seemed quite upbeat, judging by the tone of her announcement. No matter, the book was good so I'd simply be getting through it quicker. Less than sixty seconds later the cheery sod at reception announced again,

"Mr Palmer's clinic is now running an hour and a half late." There was a collective groan from the packed waiting room.

This was the opposite of time travel. The world would keep turning and we would all be here in purgatory till old age took us (for some around me it might not be that long). The amused receptionist wasn't so chuffed now; she was fending abuse from all quarters. Someone was responsible for the huge delay and unless there was a head on a spike, pronto, some of these ill and aged moaners were going to complain, officially.

Anyone who attends NHS clinics expecting to be taken on time is seriously deluded. It just takes one complex set of symptoms or a person's outcome that was unsuccessful, for a ten minute consultation to turn into a twenty minute consultation. Multiply the likelihood of this by a clinic that comprises forty people and you see why very few clinics run to time (and not because the staffs are dragging this out to avoid having lunch). I would offer the complainers of the world a spot of advice though.

Abusing your health care staff is most unwise. The receptionist you've just swore at is unlikely to put you through to see the doctor before the polite and lovely lady who sat the whole time waiting patiently. Similarly, the poor ward nurse taking a mouthful from you because you seem to think she's a slacker; she's in charge of your pain meds. Honestly, do you really want to piss her off?

If she gets "caught up" with someone else, how desperate will she be to get back to you, the mouthy moan-a-minute, when you're not being such a brave little soldier? Every other person in the clinic / ward is just as important as you are, in the eyes of staff. Single yourself out, in the wrong way, and you'll quickly diminish the "caring" part of your treatment.

Fully ninety minutes later, with a good number of pages read, it was my turn to see Mr Palmer. This guy was calm, pleasant and all business. "John and I have talked it over and it (the reconstructed neo-bladder) is definitely the way to go for such a young guy." I had been the topic of much discussion between the three consultants. This was not a routine operation by any means but these professionals were going all out to give me a quality of life that others don't get a chance at.

With a week to the deadline, nothing else really needed to be said. I thought I knew what I was in for (mistakenly) and he had all the expertise I required. After a few perfunctory questions and answers, that was it. Total face time was six minutes. He was my kind of guy; pleasant, straight and decisive. Plus I like to think I was doing my part to claw back some clinic time.

Mr Palmer reminds me very much of my lead Consultant at the Royal Infirmary, Iain. If you need your hand held and talked through a decision matrix whilst agonising over the potential risks and benefits, best go away and come back when you've come to a decision.

If however you want first rate surgery; fine, you've come to the right place (Iain Swan and Mike Palmer are like peas in a pod). Definitely, these are my kind of guys. I fully appreciated John Crooks' style of consultation that's inclusive and informative but similarly I can see the appeal of decisive, if you're ready and I'm ready then let's "crack on" type of surgeons.

D-Day Comes Around

My big birthday treat had arrived. The night had passed fitfully between fart boy across the room and the last tattered remains of my arse getting me up. I wasn't too worried about my lack of sleep; I'd be out like a light for the next eleven hours or so, once the general anaesthetic was on board.

I had skipped breakfast, not just because I had a "Nil by Mouth" sign on my bed. Very few Michelin star chefs work in the NHS canteens. Hospital food has a derisory reputation I reasoned. I was missing nothing. If I had any clue as to how long it would be before I next ate I would have kicked myself for being so glib and dismissive of the canteen staff.

Breakfast skipped, I had my "arse-less" gown and paper hat delivered by one of the nurses with a promise that one of the theatre porters was on his way to take me down to surgery. A tummy full of butterflies would be the polite way of describing how I was feeling at this point. Skull crushingly terrified might be another way of describing it.

The prospect of having internal organs permanently removed was a horrific thought. I'd been a complete individual up till to today. The disability thing had never bothered me in any way whatsoever. It had happened too young and as far as I was concerned tootling around in a wheelchair was my norm.

Both my legs were present and correct even if I didn't have the use of them, they were still attached. However having your insides scooped out and re-plumbed made me feel queasy. From today onwards I was being left with fewer parts than I was born with and ultimately there was still no guarantee of a cancer free future, despite these professionals' best efforts. My brain was flapping as fast as the butterflies' wings.

My porter duly arrived and I transferred myself onto his theatre gurney. He was clearly having a good day. He was spectacularly cheery. Astoundingly cheery, positive and winningly, hilariously fun.

What a total bastard. It was like having Krusty the clown telling endless knock-knock jokes on your way to the gallows. According to him the world was bright, the birds were singing, the sun was shining, and it was a singularly great day to be alive.

I was under a dark cloud with no positives that I could think of (where the bloody hell was Dawn's positivity when I needed it). Perhaps his was a style of portering that helped patients see that life is worth living and his effortless bonhomie took their mind off the worry of imminent surgery. I just wished he'd piss off, or at the very least be struck dumb for the remainder of the journey.

No such luck; he laughed and joked and chortled me all the way to the theatre suites and bade me "all the best. Not that you'll need it," before finally skipping off to find his next victim. Being escorted to theatre by a Dementor would have been preferable and more in keeping with my current mood.

Theatre checklists are a necessary protocol. Your wristband is checked by each staff member in turn and you're obliged to state name, date of birth and address many times. This is to make sure you are in fact who they're expecting on today's list and you don't end up with an unexpected sex change or kidney donation. I'm not in any way superstitious or doubtful of NHS staff integrity but I'd committed to memory my ten digit CHI number.

Everyone with a visit to an NHS hospital has a unique number given to avoid different hospitals creating different case note numbers for the same person. Conversely someone with a common name and the same date of birth as another sick person doesn't want to find themselves on the liver transplant list when they turn up for a vasectomy.

I rhymed off my details, including CHI number like a soldier In Stanley Kubrick's Full Metal Jacket,

"Sir, YES SIR!"

This was done at every waypoint along the conveyor belt of pre-op. Tedious certainly but completely essential. We brave few in the admission suite each had a bay, all repeating our respective personal details every few minutes.

Seven of us were here, each one of us as nervous as the next. I couldn't help looking round my fellow worriers and wondering what each person was "in for." We could have played surgical Top Trumps to pass the time.

"Length of symptoms?"

"Seven months."

"Eighteen. Beat you!"

"Ok then, estimated time in surgery?"

"Four hours."

"Ha! Eleven! In your face!"

No one here looked in the mood for a casual game, so we continued to answer the same information. I for one wanted to be on the right table with the right surgeon for the correct reason.

My semi-unique name guarantees me a certain amount of exclusivity. The only other Paul Doody I've ever heard of won

Stars in Their Eyes, singing as Marti Pellow. That couldn't have been me as I wouldn't be able to tell the difference between a C major and a Sergeant Major. (Robert Frobisher's quote from David Mitchell's Cloud Atlas)

Odd name and memorised CHI meant I definitely was in the appropriate theatre. I recognised the Anaesthetist and Mr Rajan. All were very pleasant and light-hearted. The banter between colleagues was reassuring and I was feeling positive for the first time that morning that I was in good hands. The Anaesthetist was ready to crack on with a syringe in the back of my right hand.

"All set Paul? We'll see you on the other side. Here we go."

Recovery

"Hi Paul, I'm Natalie."

It was dark. Much later the same day but clearly the operation had taken as long as expected because the clock on the opposite wall told me it was nearly nine p.m.

"How are you feeling Paul?" It was Natalie again. I had no idea how I was feeling. Fog was clouding my brain. A long day's anaesthetic had me confused and dopey.

"Are you in any pain?" She was persisting but I was struggling to come up with an answer. For one, putting the words together was a task and two; I had a mouth as dry as a camel's arse. "Try some small sips of water, that'll help." Natalie had read my befuddled brain and the water was ice cold and delicious. "Better?"

"Much." It came out like a croak from a particularly heavy smoking frog. Now with a chance to look properly at Staff Nurse Natalie, this was not a half bad way to be recovered. She was as pretty as hell; tiny, brunette with an angelic face. I could be mistaken for thinking I'd died and been woken in the afterlife (not that I go for that kind of thing).

I heartily recommend that the NHS use only the most attractive male and female recovery staff in all post-op situations. It welcomes you back to the world far more amiably than being woken by some psycho hose beast (Wayne's World quote).

"Feeling OK? Are you comfortable?" The recovery ward was like an oven. The NHS routinely heats its ward and clinic spaces to boiling point. Even my own clinic in Glasgow Royal often feels like we're working on the surface of the sun.

"I'm warm Staff Nurse, really warm." Natalie went to open a window and came back to organise my bed. "We'll bring your bed up a bit and pull back the sheets to let you cool down a little."

As the bed rose my vision suddenly reduced to tiny pin pricks of light like an old TV had been switched off and then; blackness.

Nothingness.

Back; I was back in the same room after an indiscriminate period of time. Suddenly I was awake and Natalie was pounding up and down on my chest.

"Sinus, Sinus rhythm's back!" This was someone else on the other side of the bed. A male someone had appeared without me noticing. Natalie got off. She appeared tiny but she could summon the power of the Hulk when jumping on your sternum.

"Paul? Paul! Can you hear me?" I could hear him alright, "Yeah mate, you're shouting." There was activity all around me but I wasn't too quick to pick up on what had just happened. "Have you any idea what just happened Paul?" I told him "Not a clue."

"Your heart stopped beating." He said. I had a quip ready about Natalie's face stopping any guy's heart but just couldn't seem to make the words come out. Someone else had appeared and questions were flying about me that didn't make sense.

"Have you had a heart attack before?" What kind of stupid question was that? Did he say a heart attack? Was this joker taking the piss or what? "Of course I haven't!" My indignation wasn't coming across as my voice was now down to a whisper but I couldn't figure out why. Someone called out "Bradycardia!" then; blackness.

Nothingness.

Natalie was at it again; pounding away at my chest. Pretty as she may be, I was now pissed off meeting her like this. "He's back!" someone said. The level of activity and the tone of conversation now grabbed my attention. People were stripping off my gown and attaching big grey pads to my lower left and upper right chest. Drugs were going into the drip attached to the back of my right hand.

Yet another person had arrived. This guy in particular was taking charge and asking the nursing staff lots of questions about onset, duration, resuscitation and the like. I was following none of this; my mental abilities were still affected by the anaesthetic and I was now becoming seriously distressed by their urgency.

"Paul. Is there a history of heart disease in the family?"
"No."

"Have you suffered any heart attacks in the past?"
"No."

"Do you smoke?"

Fuck sake! Not this again. I was of a mind to light up a Marlboro as soon as possible. Just to give the medical fraternity something to pin on me. "No, never smoked in my life." I wanted to give this guy a piece of my mind but it looked like I'd not have the time, if my ticker was about to give out its last tock. "How are you feeling just now?" He said.

"I'm feeling fine, mate. No worries."

This was a complete lie. I was deeply worried. There seemed to be no trigger that set these attacks off. Twice now my heart had just packed in with no warning. I was terrified that this was a degenerative condition. If this continued the cardiac muscle would begin to die off.

"What's wrong with me?" They weren't too sure which wasn't great news, judging by my current lack of rhythm. Best guess was the heart was struggling to shrug off the effects of such a long anaesthetic.

It seemed the "lub" and the "dub" of the upper and lower chambers was out of sync. If the electrical timing was even slightly off from either chamber, then the heart just stopped. It had restarted by itself a couple of times (as seen on a cardiac monitor) but twice now it had needed proper help.

Until this point I'd completely forgotten about cancer. No mean feat as it had been lurking at the back of my mind for months now. This is what it took. I was using up NHS time and resources, singlehandedly, at a furious rate. This is what the Health Service is best at though; emergency diagnosis and safe, accurate and effective treatment.

Some people complain about waiting. Others complain about the quality of treatment they receive but if you need urgent care, proper care *now*, the NHS is the envy of the developed world. One bit of me had been sorted and now another bit was broken but if I could just hang in there for long enough, this new guy would sort it out here and now.

"We can't sort this here, I'm afraid." Bugger! "We have to transfer you to the Western General where the Coronary Care Unit is." Glasgow has six main adult hospitals and one specialist paediatric hospital. Medical specialities divide up and occupy different sites spread all over the city and you may well have to visit different parts of it depending on just how much is wrong with you.

In my 23 years of service I have worked in four of the six adult hospitals. I had never, not once, been inside the Western

General. I deal solely with Ear Nose and Throat consultants, so cardiac conditions were way outside my scope of practice.

"A specialist team is going to come from the Western Coronary Care Unit in a special ambulance to transfer you back over to their ward." My new guy said. "Would it not just be easier to call me a cab?" I was being sarcastic just for effect. My delivery needed a stronger voice and perhaps a drum roll and cymbal crash. Anything to lighten the moment but this bloke had a serious irony deficiency.

"I'm not sure you appreciate quite how grave the situation is Paul." I did: and the use of "grave" was in itself ironic but he was on a roll. "Your heart is in a very weak state. You need constant monitoring by specialists to see if the anaesthetic wears off and your cardiac symptoms improve." He wasn't finished with this particular lecture. "This team are better equipped than a standard ambulance crew for cardiac care, let alone a taxi." Boy oh boy was that me told. I resolved to keep my flippant remarks to myself in future.

It was going to take a couple of hours to assemble the crew and the equipment for my transfer to the Western. I was ensconced in a single room right next to the nurse's station; all the better to keep an eye on me no doubt.

Things appeared to have settled down in the previous half hour and I was glad to have no more encounters with the brutal, beauty Natalie. A while later I was greeted with an even more comely sight: Stephanie. I could have cried with relief.

Someone clearly had called and relayed the news and she'd come running. More worrying still, the kids were here also. No point in "losing it" in front of them. Dads need to be strong and unflappable in front of their kids. No crying allowed.

Stephanie had been told on the phone that there had been some "Pauses" in my heartbeat. Once again medicine was couching the alarmist terms "Death" and "Resuscitation" into a far less threatening "Pause".

It was dark o'clock in the morning when Stephanie had been phoned so she tried in vain to get someone to come and look after the kids, who were tucked up in bed. My parents, her parents and my brother and sister-in-law were phoned but no one was answering. She was left with no alternative but to rouse them both, dress them and rush off to the hospital.

Arianne and Jonathan's faces said it all. It was painful to watch them. I must have been a fearsome sight. I had two post-op drains; one coming out of either side of my groin. A massive midline scar was covered in a dressing from the sternum down. I had cardiac pads stuck to either side of my chest in case I needed "shocked" back to life.

Multiple chest leads were attached to a monitor that was running my cardiac trace behind my head and I had two drips; one in each arm. All-in-all Dad had looked better. Thankfully Stephanie was made of sterner stuff and didn't bat an eyelid. She gave me a smile and "we kiss like we invented it." (Mirror ball by Elbow). I felt much better. Once again my overriding emotion at this point was guilt. "I'm really sorry," was all I could come up with. "I'm so sorry about this."

"So you should be." Stephanie said it with a smile. It was a gentle loving kind of smile. It was a gentle loving kind of patronising smile for the idiot who's apologising for almost dying. We held hands and reassured the kids that the worst was over. Even if we were proved wrong, it's just what had to be done. I figured if we said it in earnest to Ari and Jonny, we might just convince ourselves into the bargain.

All the staff were fabulous with our kids. It was the scariest of surroundings for children but the nurses whisked them away for a spell, to ply them both with tea and chocolate.

This gave Stephanie and I some quiet time together. It was a huge relief to hold onto her. It was almost as though my heart simply needed her there as *the* reason to keep on going.

We talked a little but it was artificially light hearted. Abject fear was uppermost in our minds but it was easier to suppress if you were pretending to be strong for one another. I could pretend to be the big guy who would bounce back from cancer plus a couple of heart attacks.

She in turn could roll her eyes and laugh at my attempts to be butch. Inside we were both like five year olds; terrified of the monster under the bed and covering our heads with metaphorical sheets.

"It's just the beast under your bed; in your closet, **in your head**," (Enter Sandman by Metallica).

The Western Trail

At some point later, the special transport arrived. Two doctors were in attendance and they were going to be with me in the back as we journeyed across the city. It wouldn't take long to get there, especially as it was still the middle of the night and traffic was minimal. The paramedic driver was to take extra care whilst getting us there as no one knew as yet what could set off the cardiac arrhythmia. No burnouts or handbrake turns were allowed, just in case it set me off on one.

The two docs were really easy going types, joking with Stephanie and I. It helped raise the mood as both resembled a couple of lost backpackers. Each had the kind of kit bag that the SAS might lug up a mountain in Wales. The hand over took an age.

Lots of special instructions were given. Lots of medications were issued. Lots of paperwork was signed and passed around between medics. Was all this for me? I was beginning to wonder if I would die of embarrassment rather than heart failure. Look at all the hassle I was causing. A last hug from my wife and kids and we were off.

I thought we might never make it. I was incredulous that any ambulance could go this slow. This guy was driving so slowly he could drive Miss Daisy. This was "funeral procession" slow. Crap, I hoped not. It was made bearable by the two docs in attendance. They were a good pair. Both well versed in black humour.

They also were watching my every breath, blink and movement. If I showed any sign of a flutter I knew they'd be all over me in a shot. I felt confident that when we arrived, if we ever arrived, I'd be well looked after. The journey was long but thankfully uneventful and we pulled up outside the Western General having shared our sickest jokes and most inappropriate stories.

The transfer to the ward in Coronary Care Unit was a complete faff. I had drains, drips and cardiac monitors to be dragged around as well as me on the ambulance gurney. Never had a lift been so tightly packed. It was like a live game of Tetris trying to get the bed and paramedic equipment plus doctors in. It wouldn't work one way so out we came to try another configuration. It took a couple of tries but we all fit in eventually.

We arrived in almost total blackness and I was transferred into the new ward's receiving room; right next to the nurse's station. It's a pole position space for the observance of the new guy. The reverse swap happened with the new staff given all the pertinent info and drugs while I recited my name and number a few times.

Finally I was afforded a proper bed and was gently slid across to my new bunk for the immediate future. Just a blonde nurse and I remained. She was moving the drips into a comfortable position and making sure the post-op drains were still working when; blackness.

Nothingness

I came back to hear her shouting "I need help here! I'M ON MY OWN HERE!" Yet another pretty nurse (just as brutal though) had saved my life and was pounding away at my sternum. I was now totally pissed off with this as a past time. I was as scared as hell and was hurting in more places at once than I thought I possessed. Strike three for team NHS. I had paused (died) properly three times and been brought back.

During each I had seen no tunnels of light, no harp music, no out of body experience. I was now more convinced than ever that I had just the one life, so live it to the full. If team NHS can keep me going I'll continue to do my utmost in every way for the benefit of those around me. "GO TEAM!"

Strike number four for the good guys. It had happened yet again. Fourth pause and fourth save for team NHS. Just a couple of hours had separated the last two attacks. It was in fact getting worse. It was increasingly likely that a temporary pacemaker was needed to keep me alive. The longer this pausing nonsense dragged on, the likelihood increased that the next "save" wouldn't work.

A temporary pacemaker would intervene and correct the pause before the heart stopped. The correction would happen in milliseconds and I wouldn't even feel it happen.

I was all for that even if the thought of an old dude's pacemaker wasn't that appealing, it was just until the heart shook off the last vestiges of anaesthetic. I'd be willing to try anything to avoid any further exposure to nurses on my chest. From first-hand experience, even if CPR was administered by the most attractive off duty supermodel / nurse, it hurts like hell.

My new ward was smaller and more intimate; being a specialist, critical unit, the nursing care was more intense and personal. Observations were often and detailed. Tracings analysed, blood pressure and pulse taken and temperature checked, all for my betterment. It was early on the second morning and I sorely needed sleep, proper sleep, not chemically induced anaesthesia. I was thoroughly done in. Sleep was not about to happen.

Hourly Obs (observations) were the newest chore to be endured. Wide awake or fast asleep you had to be checked for this, checked for that and checked for the other. I couldn't believe the difference to my body in just 48 hours. Two days ago I had felt near normal in most ways (granted with a bloody big tumour attached to my bladder) and now I was utterly beyond recognition. I had been sliced, diced, repaired and resuscitated four times. It was by far the busiest two days of my life and I thought I deserved a bit of a kip.

The majority of the new day was spent in an extended stupor. I was partially awake for the Obs but almost immediately fell back asleep when the nurse / doctor had left. I had been personally introduced to a whole new team of nurses and doctors but was unable to process or recall anything that had been said.

I was a bag of flesh and bone whose owner had taken a well-earned leave of absence. My poor body didn't know if it was "shot, fucked, powder-burnt or snake bit," (a quote from Robin Williams' Good Morning, Vietnam). I had slept a good portion of the day away so that by visiting time I was much more conscious of the environment.

Stephanie was back, this time with my parents and no children in tow. After I had been taken from Gartnavel, Stephanie took the kids back home for a couple of hours sleep. She then got them back up at their usual time and packed the pair off to school. No special day off for our kids; it was routine as normal so as to keep them focused on the mundane.

Stephanie was looking as fresh as a daisy. Remarkable on so little sleep and maximum stress but she is made of different stuff from the rest of us mere mortals. Anne and Eddie were their usual bright and positive selves. My parents also come from a different stock than the norm. They are the epitome of "Capable in the Face of Adversity!" Coping strategies must be hard-wired into these people as the collective story of their lives reads like a partnership forged in turmoil.

Catholic boy meets Protestant girl and they fall in love. Cast out by their respective families during a time where religions are forbidden to mix, they seek refuge with a sympathetic aunt. They promptly get married in a small ceremony with little family in attendance. She finds out she's pregnant with their first child (that would be me). His sister suddenly requires a ground-breaking risky kidney transplant op and he volunteers as a donor. The transplant is a success for both parties. His wife delivers a second child at full-term which is still-born. A year later the first child runs into traffic at age three and is a paraplegic for life. She finds out that she is pregnant again whilst caring for the disabled child and he now has to urgently rush off down to the south of England as his closest brother dies.

It goes on and on like this and yet these two remarkable people manage to stay together weathering each new storm whilst raising my brother Simon and me in a perfectly normal childhood.

Eddie had donated a kidney to his sister in 1969 which was still ground breaking and terrifyingly risky at that point: braver still when you have your first child on the way. The first NHS kidney transplant had been done only nine years earlier.

Michael Woodruff in Edinburgh Royal Infirmary transplanted a kidney between adult twins. The operation was a complete success for each of the twins, due in part to the absence of rejection with the recipient of the organ.

Eddie still plods along to this day with his remaining kidney, regularly flushing the poor thing through with good chardonnay. His sister Rita thrived for two and a bit decades post op before falling foul of the body's own rejection mechanisms. It was a huge gamble in its day and paid massive dividends.

It's only when you piece the significant events of their life together do you realise my parents remain positive in the face of a mutant hybrid of Greek tragedy and black comedy.

If they were surprised by my appearance, they didn't show it. Stephanie had seen the look I was sporting earlier so was unfazed. This was the time of maximum stress yet we were all smiles. Not denial in any way, no one was deluding themselves but people who have lived through tough times are harder to upset than normal, that's all.

Ward staff were re-introduced to us with platitudes like "he gave us quite a scare", "he's in good hands" and "what's he like?" It was the light-hearted banter which people affect in your presence as though you posed only a minor inconvenience.

My cosy new room was a godsend compared to my proposed four bedded ward in Gartnavel. I even had a TV with a remote control all to myself no less. No Cartoon Network, no Disney XD or worse, Loose Women. I could lie back and doze between repeats of Top Gear. Bliss.

The only fly in the ointment was the impending temporary pacemaker insertion. This is normally done under local anaesthetic and I was not looking forward to it.

Pace Setter

I was taken to theatre in my own bed this time due to the fact I was attached to more lights and wiring than a Christmas tree. There was the surgeon, the blonde nurse from the night before and also a Radiologist to provide imaging for the insertion of the pacing wire into my heart. The procedure should in theory take no more than thirty minutes in tops.

We're now at a developmental point in cardiac research that a paltry half hour is all it takes to artificially time the series of events that keep each one of us alive. Famously, Christiaan Barnard carried out the first heart transplant in 1967 in Capetown. There is a superb display in the Glasgow Science Centre which details the ground breaking procedure.

A year after the South African pioneering surgery, Donald Ross and a team of eighteen performed the NHS' first heart transplant in the National Heart Hospital in London. It was the 3rd May 1968 and was the tenth operation to be done anywhere in the world. The NHS has always been at the tip of innovation

With a local anaesthetic in the left side of my neck the pacing wire went down my left internal jugular vein on its way across the body to the right atrium. At this point the surgeon (in theory) tries to create a loop of wire in the top right chamber by pinning it against the muscle wall and then rotates the wire so it flips into the lower ventricle via the tricuspid valve.

As easy as that sounds, we were having no such bloody luck. I was causing this surgeon heart ache in cardiac theatre. Time and again the poor sod got the loop pinned against the atrial wall above the valve, rotated the wire and "Boink" it came straight back out.

"Scientific progress goes Boink" (Calvin and Hobbes by Bill Waterson)

Fifty long torturous minutes later and we were finally in business. Wire in the lower chamber but still the tricky voltage and timing of the pulse had yet to be set. This was the oddest most unpleasant sensation I have ever felt. As the pacing was set, suddenly your heart hammered in your chest. Adjustments made then "Bam" your heart was pounding again with no warning.

Over and over we went so the electrode would be timed beautifully to intervene if the ventricle synchronised poorly. This little wire may be distressing but it was quite literally a lifesaver.

Many minutes passed and at last it was all in place and the pacing wire was physically stitched into my neck to avoid an accidental tug and then thoroughly covered in a dressing. Throughout the procedure I was asked time after time if I needed a break as we could time-out and let me rest. This was very considerate but I wanted this done and dusted so urged the surgeon to crack on and just get it over with. Now that it was over, I was knackered. I'd done nothing but lie with my head canted to the right for over an hour but I was now absolutely wrecked.

The next few days were pure recovery. Not just from the cardiac perspective but from the major surgery. I was immobile at the neck from pacing, pinned from the waist with surgical drains and one arm had a constant drip with fluid and glucose. In short I was going nowhere. Visitors began appearing at intervals over the days that followed. There were lots of worried faces and stoic "keep your chin up" pleasantries.

Stephanie's parents, Bill and Christine got their first look at me in cardiac care. Not until weeks later they openly confessed that they were certain their daughter was destined to be a widow, judging by how I looked. I was in pain, certainly. The morphine was controlling the worst of it but inside I had my first really positive thoughts for recovery. The imminent danger had now passed and all that was needed from here on in was time.

Dawn began visiting the new unit after her shift. However, loaded with new and interesting meds, I had missed her visits a couple of times. She'd been making the effort to find me in a new hospital and I'd done her the honour of being out-for-the-count. How charming of me.

Other unexpected visitors began making daily journeys to my bedside. Mr Crooks and Mr Rajan were fitting in a personal visit to me, regardless of their packed schedule. This could be for one of two reasons. Either they were genuinely worried about my general well-being or conversely they were desperate to make sure I didn't die and ruin a full day's hard work into the bargain.

I was touched by the sentiment either way. One consultant would wash and alco-gel his hands, check the post op drains and wound, ask the nursing staff about fluid balance and generally reassure me that the surgery couldn't have gone better. These men went out of their way to travel each day to see me and I appreciated the effort and time each gave.

A comfortable routine established itself over the next week. Lots of quiet convalescence coupled with afternoon visiting, evening visiting and Top Gear in between. Stephanie was looking after the kids during the school week off, trying desperately to keep them entertained (distracted) and visiting as often as possible. She was organising the rest of the family; putting a schedule in place to avoid too many visitors at the same time and none at others.

She was keeping a great many plates spinning all at once (she had also started a new national NHS job to boot) and was still able to act like she was pleased to see me. The stress must have been immense. The hardest part of my day was if the TV remote was just out of reach. Stephanie's head at this point must have been a whirlwind of outwardly calm organisation during the day and lonely late night terror.

"I'm living in cloud cuckoo land. And this just feels like spinning plates." (Spinning Plates by Radiohead)

In idle moments I wondered how I'd be remembered, if things didn't work out. Would my passing go unnoticed, bar a eulogy and a family piss up? Or would it go the other way? No one would want to be remembered for their flaws after all.

"To Paul Doody!" A glass gets raised in my name in an anonymous bar.

"Who are we drinking to?"

"Paul Doody. You must have heard of him."

"Nope. I don't know who that was."

"You've got to be kidding. This is Paul Doody we're talking about. He was one hell of a guy. Kind to a fault, funnier than any comedian and he could turn his hand to anything. He could fix cars, lift weights, play drums and repair computers. Not only was he a hell of a guy but he was an attentive father, a loving husband, hardworking, loyal and honest."

"He sounds like a superb all round good guy. I'm sorry I never met him."

"I never met him either. I married his bloody widow."

After a week had passed since my birthday, the consultant cardiologist thought that it was the right time to remove the temporary pacemaker. It had kept me going like clockwork and the majority of the anaesthetic should have metabolised by now (residuals can last up to a month). I was perfectly happy to have it out. Lifesaving it may be but it was deeply inconvenient. I wasn't able to move much, turn over without help or relieve the constant pressure on my neck. It had done a terrific job but I was now seriously pissed off with it. The CCU staff had been attentive to a fault. Who could ask for more?

To take out the pacemaker took three people. A senior staff nurse, a junior nurse and a student nurse. It was a delicate procedure requiring skilful coordination to avoid cata-strophic blood loss. They began by cutting the stitches holding the sheath of the wire to my neck. Next the pacemaker wire was removed, the easy bit. Then the sheath had to be removed and pressure immediately applied by the second person to the jugular while the third watched to make sure there was no loss of consciousness.

All this had to be done in one fluid swift motion or the room was about to be redecorated in a fine red mist. They were totally ace at it, making it look as routine as tying shoe-laces. The pressure applying nurse had to stay in place for ten minutes with just the right amount of push. Too much and she'd throttle me and too little, she'd resemble a butcher's apron. Clotting by the ten minute point should have sealed the jugular. Go platelets!

My only gripe (and it's a minor one), was that in removing the initial dressings they had removed half my beard with it. They gave me a unilateral face strip wax. I've had a beard non-stop since my late teens. Not a grubby long soup-strainer you understand. A nice trim shaped beard, without which I look like a round faced child.

Stephanie forbade me from shaving it off years ago as I look "wrong" without it. I certainly looked "wronger" with only half of it left. I uttered no words of complaint as you can hardly moan to the people saving your life that they left you with a wonky face. But they did.

Freedom to look around was a relief as was the end of the drip in the right arm. I could look to the left. I could massage my sore neck and scratch my arse at the same time. Small wins, for sure but it was a big difference in terms of mobility even though the drains were still attached and draining away. I could wash unassisted for the first time in days and came upon an unwelcome shock. My bollocks were huge, massive, swollen to the size of party balloons.

I was the living embodiment of "Buster Gonad" from Viz. I knew from the early consultations that the surgery was predominately from the abdomen but the re-plumbing would also involve coming at it from "down below". I still wasn't prepared for *this*.

These nuts might not be big enough to carry around in a wheelbarrow but if the swelling didn't go down, I'm sure they'd tuck into my socks. At visiting that night I regaled the family that my balls were so big it took both hands to wash just one of them. I meant it as a boast but they took it as a joke. It was the first levity we'd had in days. (Buster Gonad; "the boy with the unfeasibly large testicles" from Viz magazine)

The morning of the 13th February and the new topic of discussion was just how soon I could be transferred back to Gartnavel to the intended post-op Urology ward. I had been in cardiac care for almost a week and couldn't fault the attention I'd had since the opening drama. I was off the drip and onto oral painkillers instead and whilst taking the last in a long line of meds, the final tablet stuck in my throat.

I coughed hard to dislodge it then; black.

Nothingness

The now all too familiar activity greeted me on resus. Hopes had now been dashed. It wasn't going away. I was crushed physically and metaphorically. Urgent talks were now under way to see just how soon a permanent pacemaker could be inserted. Consultants consulted and nurses set every conceivable lifesaving apparatus within an arm's length of my bed.

A permanent pacemaker had to be ordered up and a consultant found to insert it A.S.A.F.P (ASAP only more so). After many phone calls my name had been force added to the end of a surgeon's list tomorrow in Glasgow Royal Infirmary.

This was the soonest available slot in the city. I would literally be going home. The transport was ordered up again and I sat forlorn at the thought of yet another procedure, albeit on my own turf but just as unwelcome as a pair of huge balls.

Keeping the Pace

Another journey took place more in keeping with the Reverend W Awdry stories. A gradual saunter to the Royal Infirmary took treble the time it should have or could have, if I'd been allowed to drive the ambulance. Stephanie had left the Western Infirmary at the same point the ambulance had and was camped outside ward 43 with an "about bloody time" look on her face. Settling in took minutes and once again we were introduced to a new team in yet another new ward.

Being on home ground was no consolation at all. I hadn't expected bunting and parades but the emotional lift at coming home that I was expecting didn't arrive. Needing a pacemaker at 43 years of age was momentous. Stephanie's Dad had one fitted but he was in his sixties, so it didn't seem such an odd occurrence. I looked and felt a million years old since developing a dodgy ticker.

"It's not the years honey. It's the mileage." (Indiana Jones to Marion in Raiders of the Lost Ark)

The new ward was typical for Glasgow Royal: hot. How the staff did manual handling in these temperatures was beyond me. It was like a furnace. I wasn't allowed any food due to the planned op the next day but I was allowed ice cubes. I developed an obsession with ice. Just holding it in my mouth was heaven. I would hold it to my forehead. I would rest it on my eyes. I would let it drip, drip, drip on my chest. The heat was a physical force.

If anyone asked if there was anything I needed the answer was always: ice. You could re-sink the Titanic with the quantity of ice I got through. It was now the 13th February and in the days since my birthday I'd had very little to eat. Most of my sustenance had been in drip form. Lurching from procedure to procedure my nil-by-mouth status had been seldom interrupted. Hunger didn't even factor in the equation as far as I was concerned. I was getting by on a diet of stress and frozen water. Later that afternoon and for no apparent reason I had another "pause". This one self-corrected and the heart continued to thrum and I came to after just a few seconds as though nothing had happened. Stephanie had hit the buzzer as soon as the cardiac monitor had signalled an alarm but by the time the nurse had appeared, I'd come around and was back in the room.

I was living on borrowed time and my procedure was late on tomorrow afternoon's list. Would I be able to hold on long enough? I was driving myself crazy with the urgency of it all. I could have cried out in frustration.

Dawn visited that same evening and I was possibly the worst host on the planet. This ward was just upstairs from our clinic so she was much less inconvenienced in catching me here. I was glad to see her for sure but nothing she or Stephanie could say would help with my feeling of dread. They were trying really hard to be light-hearted, positive and chatty but I couldn't even force myself to join in. I simply wanted to fast-forward to the same time tomorrow night when it would all be over.

Very late on in the day, the two women in my life were gone with heavy hearts when another visitor arrived; Adam. My mate had heard through the grapevine about me being on home turf and had decided to try for a religious conversion while I was at my weakest (I'm only half joking). He spent some time saying extremely nice things about my personality, my endurance, strength of character and the sheer numbers of people relying on my recovery.

As a counsellor he was putting perspectives in front of me that I had been neglecting. I had allowed myself to turn inward and become less aware of the wider reasons why I had to survive and endure. He asked if he was allowed to say a short prayer at my bedside and who was I to argue? This man is a credit to his profession.

A very long and lonely night passed. Sleep was elusive but I must have drifted off in the early hours of the 14th. At around seven am the ward became a hive of activity. Routine Obs, breakfasts (not for me) and showers are all due before the shift change at eight. I was simply an observer this morning.

My procedure was going to be later this afternoon. All I had to do was wait. I have never been good at waiting. Less so when I'm watching a clock with my breath held, praying my turn would come sooner than expected. It didn't come any quicker for all my wishes.

A porter arrived at around two thirty (two thirty three exactly. I was glued to the clock). This guy was more my kind of porter. Quiet. Not like that cheery bastard in Gartnavel. The theatres were close and it took no time getting there. Waiting in turn in pre-op I had a glimmering of hope that this might be *it*. Maybe, just maybe it would be the end to "pausing".

Dying didn't suit me too well and let's be honest; I'd hung on thus far. In total my heart had stopped eleven times. Five of those I had needed lots of assistance. My NHS had now dragged me back from the abyss multiple times. How would you express the gratitude to those involved?

Words surely aren't enough? The gratitude extends much farther than personal gain. The benefits ripple and extend through to your wife, children, parents, friend and ultimately all those lives you touch every day. I'm indebted and will pay it forward.

At last it was my turn. The team were already set up with my pacemaker sealed in a sterile container. The wire placement was extremely quick in comparison to the temporary version. The consultant had it in place in one fluid attempt. What a pro.

The difficulty in this op was sighting the processor under the left clavicle in a pouch which needs to be carved out above the muscle but below the skin. Local anaesthetic aside there was a lot of violent, uncomfortable pushing and pulling to fit the battery and control unit under my left collar bone.

The pacemaker itself is a blunt teardrop shaped pebble. It's approximately three inches by two and once it was connected to the pacing wire the unpleasant timing and voltage was set. Job done; the total time for this one had been a paltry thirty minutes. The same time you'd wait for a pizza delivery. I was now a repaired and relieved man. "Pauses" were now a full stop. I was so relieved in fact that I openly, un-self-consciously wept. The theatre staff must have thought I was some kind of drama queen but I didn't mind.

On the 14th February 2013 the cardiac team in Glasgow Royal Infirmary finally fixed a broken heart in order for me to hand it back to its rightful owner. Happy Valentine's day to Stephanie and sorry I didn't get you a card.

R and R

On the move again, yet another ambulance was requested to transport me over to Gartnavel's Urology ward 6. I commented at this point that the NHS should have some form of "air miles" for frequent flyers. I had been in so many transports by now my credits could have got me half way around the world.

The biggest difference to this journey was speed. We positively rocketed back up Great Western road. No need this time to fanny around worrying about pathetic, peripatetic Paul. It felt like NASCAR compared to the Thomas the Tank transport of the previous ambulances.

The familiar edifice of Gartnavel General Hospital hove into view and I hoped this would be the final move. Rest and recuperate was all I had to accomplish. On the protracted journey I began wondering if histology had been done on my tissue samples in the lab. This would be the biggest cloud over the horizon for my long term future.

Messrs Crooks and Rajan had removed all sorts of lymph nodes in various locations to assess the extent and the spread of the cancer. Now my status had changed from critical to stable I could afford to think slightly longer term than the end of each day.

If any one of the lymph nodes came back positive for disease then the future was bleak. It meant the tumour was already elsewhere, spread body-wide within the lymphatic system and multiplying exponentially.

If however the lab found no spread into the tissues then it was site specific and all cleared by the surgeon's skill. Wouldn't that be something? These were truly lottery odds and I was interrupted mid-thought by arriving at Gartnavel.

I was taken to the fifth floor, left out of the lifts and along a familiar corridor. Back to my starting point all those days ago and not exactly looking forward to finding who my dormitory mates would be. No one as it turned out. I had a single room, en-suite shower and a full window with an eastern view. My luck had finally turned.

This was magnificent luxury. Once again the strange mixes of seventies gloss work and uber-technical bed persisted but not having to abide others' snoring was splendid.

"See the luck I've had; could make a good man turn bad." (Please, please, please by The Smiths)

Barring catastrophe this bed would be mine for a few weeks more and then home. Introductions lasted most of the day as people came and went about the caring profession. I had developed a minor celebrity status. "Oh you're the guy they're all talking about" sums up the comments. I was the talk of the Steamie.

One of the male nurses even described me as "the guy who refused to die". He also said that the shift hand over report had never, not once, taken so long. It took them thirty minutes just to cover my history and resuscitations thus far. I tried to give all the credit to the recovery team and CCU but the hushed tones seemed to be describing some bulletproof super-spaz.

The main nurse on my side of the ward was a woman called Barbara. She was the epitome of an NHS "Matron" of old. She was exceptionally kind to me but there was a steel edge to her voice. Barbara had been in nursing for a very long time and was well versed in the "care component" and new modern NHS systems. We hit it off straight away and had similar views on a great many things.

As reunions go, none were more heartfelt than that evenings. Stephanie visited and brought my wheelchair. The ward had locked it away and put a patient wrist band on it with my details. No ordinary chair; it's bespoke, light and able to turn on a dime. I now had independence, freedom, mobility, liberty (ok you get it by now). Getting in and out was still a huge faff though. I had surgical drains on my left groin and stents draining urine on my right. I was determined to get around under my own steam.

Laying the drains and catheters on my lap I could carefully shuffle my butt to the side of the bed, transfer to the chair and then hang the bags of fluid on the brake levers. After just a few minutes moving round the room I was out of puff. It was shocking how little stamina I could muster. A great many hours in the gym had been undone in just a couple of weeks. Superman I was not. Delighted I definitely was. Being immobile was hugely frustrating and now I was up and about I was beaming with joy.

Stephanie had also brought my second most important possession. My phone. More than just telecommunication it is my music player, a book reader, a TV and a repository of movies I had prepared in advance of the surgery. Until now I had been preoccupied with simply getting through to the end of each day but now I could occupy myself and avoid watching the clock slowly ticking around.

My phone provider was 3 and I had an unlimited data contract which I planned to exploit ruthlessly. It was also a source of comfort. People now knew I was contactable and a wealth of goodwill came flooding through via text and social media. Posts on Facebook that evening kept friends and extended family informed and best wishes were pouring in from the other side of the planet.

The next day dawned spectacularly. The eastern view gave me a clear sun-up that would have inspired the great poets. Kelvingrove was back lit in orange and gold. Glasgow's nickname is Raintown though there was no sign of it this morning. The morning kept getting better and better. I was allowed breakfast. It was perhaps the best breakfast I've ever tasted. Fruit, toast with marmalade and coffee. My first coffee in weeks was like ambrosia.

I often joke that I like my coffee the same way I like my women; hot and bitter. This particular brew came in a huge bowser and was dispensed by a health care assistant into an oversize china mug. It was very hot and extremely bitter. The caffeine surge was something to experience. I never "feel" the caffeine in most espressos but since I hadn't had any for weeks I was now buzzing like fluorescent lights.

With a little freedom to move I did my best impression of Bambi, wobbling and shuffling around the room and decided to try and spruce myself up a bit. Barbara politely offered a towel and a razor. There was a slight edge to the suggestion as opposed to an offer. It wasn't till I looked in a hand-held mirror (the other being way above my head height), that I realised she was being less than subtle.

Short hair, sunken cheeks, pale blue eyes with dark bags below, crazy wild man beard with a big patch missing, newly punctured neck and freshly stitched shoulder where the pacemaker sat. I looked like a maniac from a horror movie. I blunted the first razor and asked for another. The second one lasted no time at all. In total it took four disposable blades to get the Chewbacca chops smooth.

I looked like a new man or a hastily sewn together old man if you prefer. Initial foray over, it was back to bed and get stuck into some books. What with reading, afternoon nap, afternoon visiting, dinner, evening visit and TV streamed on the phone; that was the first full day in Urology. It had flown by. This same routine continued for the next few days and the visitors (Mr Crooks included) became more and more animated and relaxed as they could see me building strength.

On the Sunday afternoon one of the staff nurses had been tasked with removing the staples from the surgical wound. This was no mean feat. The wound started below my sternum, went straight down, detoured around my belly button then ended right at my pubic bone. In total forty two staples came out (42 is the answer to life, the universe and everything according to author Douglas Adams). Not all came willingly, some needed serious effort to prise out. This was being added to my "list of hellish experiences best avoided in the future". The list was growing by the day.

The wound now felt irritable and nippy. I was uncomfortable in any position, sitting or lying. Stephanie brought the kids for afternoon visiting and even she could see I was unable to concentrate because of the pain. I was moving around in the chair but even little minor movements were sending stabbing pains through my abdomen. Once they had gone I decided I would just spend the rest of the day propped up in bed, not moving. I now had a system for getting from the chair to the bed with all the tubes and bags. One leg up, tubes on the lap, slide the butt onto the edge of the bed then recline and pull the other leg along with you.

Just as I lay back an almighty burning sensation erupted through my core. I fell back gasping in agony. Something was definitely not right. I couldn't move. I felt as though someone was holding a red hot poker to my stomach. I flailed around trying to sit up but I had no muscle control down either side. I was drenched in sweat after just a few seconds. I needed help, urgently.

I could reach the bedside unit but it only had my phone on it. The buzzer for the nurses was way out of reach. I couldn't see what had happened but the camera on my phone would show me. I shakily unlocked and navigated the menu to get the camera going and snapped off a couple of photos. What I saw was a sight from hell. My wound had completely ripped open.

You could see right inside me!

My stomach resembled like a gore soaked potato. Split right down the middle, bright red with darker viscera beneath. I was appalled, stunned and morbidly fascinated by the lack of blood. I wasn't bleeding at all. It was butcher's shop horrific sight.

I tried to push the two sides back together. The pain was incredible. I was horrified to touch it and panic was building that my insides were pushing up and out from below. I was panting and gasping like a marathon runner. I began to scream out for a nurse; a wounded, terrified cry for help.

The staff nurse who came running took one look and simply said "Oh Paul, no!" She took immediate charge, buzzed for assistance and paged the on-call registrar. Strong pain meds were given then sterile dressing packs were soaked in saline and packed into and around the wound. I was shaking violently in shock and soaked in sweat. I was incoherently mumbling to myself not to panic, don't panic, don't panic. I was not listening to my own advice and panicking wildly. The doctor arrived.

What followed was a scene taken straight from a horror movie. He washed and gloved up. He then pushed his hands down into the wound to test the extent of the tear. His fingers disappeared all the way in. My eyes grew large at the sight of his hand inside my stomach.

He said "I have to see if the tear extends into the sheath," as both hands pulled and pushed way inside. I couldn't turn away. I was transfixed. I shook and panted for what felt like an eternity.

"Your wound has dehisced completely I'm afraid" He began.

"Dehisced means…"

"I KNOW WHAT IT FUCKING MEANS!" I would later apologise for my behaviour.

"YOU CAN SEE INSIDE ME FROM ACROSS THE ROOM!" I had totally lost it and the stress of the event had pushed me over the edge.

"FIX THIS! FIX IT! FIX IT! FIX IT!"

I couldn't help myself. A rational distant part of my brain could objectively see the mess I'd become and I later reflected on how little control I had on my hysteria.

"We will. I'm going to go and make some phone calls."

He left and Barbara appeared to try and calm me down. She stood with me holding my hand and tried to talk sense to me. It would be ok. It would be stitched back up. It would all be fine once the docs did their bit. It'll be sorted soon, don't worry.

She kept this soothing litany up for a long time and gradually the rational part of my personality began to assert itself once more. It helped that the pain killers were having an effect. More importantly I could no longer see the bloody edges of my rent stomach. As disturbing as it felt, it looked far worse.

I tried to take control of my hyperventilation. The shaking became shivering due to the cold, wet dressings. I was able to comprehend, at last, that this was eminently fixable. It wasn't the end of the world; just another bump in the road. The mad panic was subsiding and I was able to speak coherently for the first time. I thanked Sister for being so patient with me. I was rewarded with a big cuddle.

I had to phone Stephanie. Now that I was under control, I had to let her know what had happened and to put off this evening's visitors. No one would want to see this. I was wrong; one person did. A difficult conversation followed and I pretended to be calm and unperturbed. Nothing was further from the truth. A short while later my visitor arrived. Simon. He had decided that I needed company in a time of need. He was calm, supportive but best of all, hilarious.

"Fucking paper cut mate."

"Did one of those the last time I shaved."

"Forget about sutures. What you need is gaffer tape, bud. I've got some in the car."

Simon works for the Scottish Ambulance Service and his patch takes in some of the less affluent areas of Lanarkshire. There is nothing which can surprise this boy. He has seen much worse than what I had on offer. He was just what I needed at that precise moment; perspective.

We sat and talked. He did extremely well at keeping my mind off the situation at hand. He told some gory stories and we laughed until the registrar came back. They shook hands and Simon said,

"Simon?"

The registrar said "Yes?"

Simon said "Simon!"

The registrar said "Yes!"

Simon said "No, Simon. It's me. Simon!"

I was clearly messed up on pain medication. I was lost all of a sudden.

Simon said "You're Simon. You were the attending at A&E in Hairmyres and I was in one of your ambulance crews."

The registrar's light bulb lit up above his head.

"Simon? Of course, you're Simon." I was now wishing I was a Simon. They had a boy's reunion of sorts, recounting some of the funnier and grosser sights they had seen in East Kilbride's main accident and emergency hospital.

I hated to interrupt but presumably Simon (the registrar version) had returned with some news and not just for the "craic". I left it as long as was polite, considering my insides were nearly on the outside. Simon (the registrar one) had spoken to his senior consultant and they were convening an emergency theatre suite and a team in order to repair me with high tension sutures.

The only issue was timing. It could take a couple of hours to assemble the theatre staff; nurses, anaesthetist and the consultant himself would have to travel in from home. Hastily arranged overtime was the order of the day, this being a Sunday. Simon (the brother one) was allowed to stay with me until the doctors and nurses had arrived and scrubbed in.

Once again I was preparing for yet another anaesthetic and yet another procedure. I dug deep and harked back to my favourite method of dispelling self-pity. What the hell could be worse than this? What if it was one of the kids? Surely that would be miles worse. If Arianne was the seriously ill or Jonny was hospitalised, I'd be agonise and impotent. For sure, that would be worry and stress and helplessness on an apocalyptic scale. So let's pretend you volunteered in their stead, that you were given an elemental choice in the matter.

Feel better? Actually yes; much better. In mentally fabricating control in a stressful situation it suddenly felt less sinister. If only the option actually existed for those parents of extremely sick children. Parents would be leaping at the chance to swap with their kids. I bet Alison and Bobby had wished many times for a parallel universe in which they could swap with Ewan. I played pretend that this was my parallel universe and I had opted in voluntarily. This helped greatly.

It was almost eleven pm when the porter arrived to take me to theatre. No more glib wishing for a cheery porter versus a dour porter. Any able bodied soul with a vague sense of direction of where we were going would do. I was no longer childishly fussy about such things. As long as I arrived in pre-op without anything falling out of my abdomen I'd not complain.

Simon, (the brother one) and I shared a manly hand shake and off we went. Pre-op was like a ghost town when the porter and I arrived. This being late on a Sunday night, I was their only customer. Two theatre nurses were ready for us and the necessary safety checks were run through, just to make sure I wasn't about to undergo a late night lung transplant.

I was taken into the theatre suite and recognised Simon's (the registrar one's) boss. It was Mr Hendry. He was a well-known surgeon in both Glasgow Royal Infirmary and Gartnavel General. I'm on a nodding relationship with a great many professionals in the Royal. My office is on a direct route from the outpatient clinics to the canteen.

My clinic is number seven, next to the lifts and clinics one through six are just a fire door away. I addressed Mr Hendry by name and profusely thanked the rest of the team for coming in to fix me. He gave me a quizzical look until Simon explained where I worked. I wasn't expecting to be recognised as I was missing my defining feature. It was back in my room, parked next to my bed. Mr Hendry and Simon assured me that once they were done I'd be unable to open my new stitches with anything less than bolt cutters.

So far my R and R had less to do with rest and recuperation and more to do with ripping and repairing. The familiar sensation of the anaesthetic delivery took place and my final medicated and stuporous thought before going under was:

"While he was down there, I should have asked him to sew in a six pack!"

Re-recovery

I came round at dark o'clock in the morning. The room was pitch-black save for a monitor's glow. The familiar beep of an Alaris was the only sound. I craned this way and that but it was pointless. There was nothing to see. I tentatively felt around under the sheet, just to make sure the job had been done. The dressing over the wound was light and I could feel the sutures below. They had zipped me up alright. It was as tight as Victorian corsetry.

"Omnishambles" is a word first used by the swearing enthusiast Malcolm Tucker in Armando Iannucci's The Thick of It. That was the perfect word for how I was feeling at that point. There was no part of me that didn't hurt directly or in sympathy. The stomach had been done twice, two types of pacemaker, groin drain, stents and jugular wounds. I was a total omnishambles.

I was struggling to take deep breaths. My stomach was now so tight it felt as though my kidneys had been relocated just below my armpits. Mr Hendry, Simon and the theatre team had done me proud. I was whole again. Flashbacks to the tear made feel queasy so I kept my mind occupied by feeling around the bed. I found the call button on a stand to my right. I gave it a stab. A nurse arrived and switched on a lamp to my left.

"Hello stranger."

"Natalie!" A guy could get used to this. The recovery process is all the more rewarding when the nursing staffs are easy on the eye. She fussed around me and sourced more ice cold water. Natalie set about doing the essential obs and we got to talking about my last recovery, weeks ago.

"Thanks for such a crap night shift."

I apologised for all the hassle I'd caused but I did casually remind her that it wasn't a bundle of laughs for me either. She'd been kept up to date on my progress by the medical staff but was astounded it had all gone wrong again. That made two of us.

The doctors figured that the dehisced wound was most likely caused by poor heart function. Since my heart perfusion had been so poor, there had been little or no real healing going on. As soon as the staples had been removed, there was nothing holding me together.

We talked a little longer and I had some pain killers. Natalie suggested I get some actual sleep as I wouldn't be going anywhere till early afternoon. That sounded like a good idea. I reclined myself into a flat position and assured her that I would behave this time around.

"You'd better!" Remembering how strong she was last time, I sincerely hoped so.

The morning brought a light breakfast; easy to digest and not much of it. I felt as if a car had parked on my middle, so a little food felt like a lot. Nurses appeared regularly to turn me off to one side or the other in order to relieve pressure. I wasn't allowed to sit upright but had to remain as horizontal as possible. I was still the only occupant of this particular recovery room. No company and no distractions meant for a long, boring morning. My first distraction arrived just after twelve pm.

Dawn. She was due to attend a manager's meeting at half past one and had left Glasgow Royal early to visit. I was never happier to see her. She gave me the gentlest hug she could manage and a "what the fuck" look. I recounted the previous day's highlights and by her expression I was once again the most pitiful excuse for a bloke ever.

I now was getting looks from people reserved for injured puppies. We talked about the latest catastrophe. I laughed at her having to attend all these meetings in my place. We simply passed the time and pondered how long it would be before I healed and got back to normality. She and I both hoped it wouldn't be too long.

My extended convalescence would directly affect Dawn. Not least because her mate was extremely ill but she was also "acting up" in my absence. All the managerial duties were allocated to her as well as a full clinical load. Dawn was put temporarily in charge of Glasgow Royal Audiology. Paid better to do the extra work but under intense pressure to keep two sets of duties balanced at the same time.

We talked shop for over an hour to maintain the illusion of normality. By all accounts our department was in good hands. Dawn was putting systems in place, so that the remaining people were given greater responsibilities. She ran through a couple of the new ways, checking what I thought about them. She was deliberately involving me and it felt great to be normal, even if it was just for a little while.

The point came where she had to go and face the powwow on the fourth floor. Another gentle hug goodbye and I wished her luck with the other team leads. She bloody well needed it. I preferred to stay here and take my chances with hospital acquired infections.

The second pair of distractions appeared soon after. My parents arrived shortly after Dawn had left. More pitiful looks ensued and lots of "You don't do things by half!" comments. I could tell the feeling of helplessness was hitting them hard. If all parents want to protect their kids from harm, I was realising age isn't a factor. Even though I was a strapping man of forty three, I was sensing that my Mother and Father would have climbed any mountain to prevent all this happening to their son. My Mum and Dad were thinking of me in exactly the same way I thought of Ari and Jonny. I found it really amusing to be thought of in those terms.

We passed the time with family gossip and messages passed through them to me, from well-wishers. Not long into their visit a porter arrived to take me back to the Urology ward and my own room. It was odd to think of it as "my room" as I'd only spent a few days there but it held my belongings, such as they were.

As a group we arrived back in the ward in no time and my parents set about putting everything within arms' reach. Suitably comfortable and contactable, visiting was over for the afternoon. For the second time in twelve hours I promised I'd try hard to be good and avoid any further drama.

I went about informing my nearest and dearest. I switched on the Samsung and phoned Stephanie at work. She was planning to visit later and I wanted to tell her all was well and whole again. Simon had to make do with a text as he can't answer his mobile at work. Once I'd covered the in-laws it was time to settle down and bide my time till evening visiting.

Stephanie was clearly relieved to see me in one piece with her own eyes. I had heaped stress upon stress on her and the family. No cracks were showing yet but how much more could she endure? We sat as a family; she and I holding hands, chatting and the two kids sat and watched TV on the phone. Arianne was acting as normal and as chatty as usual. Jonny was a different matter. He was quiet and distant. It was affecting him as the youngest. He was less able to process the stress and worry, being only eight years old.

Jonathan idolised his Dad. Jonny's Dad had huge muscles. Jonny's Dad could fix anything. Jonny's Dad was excellent on the Playstation. Now Jonny's Dad was suddenly fragile and grey and weak and mortal and Jonny was worried he was losing him. It was written all over his wee face. I was breaking his heart in being so unwell. He had big expectations that I was failing, literally, to live up to. Where was the bomb-proof, muscle-bound fixer of cars now?

Stephanie was reassured at this visit that I was sewn up tight. Arianne was glad I was well enough to even cope with a great big bear-hug. Jonathan was glum and clearly glad when time was up. When they'd gone a reality check was in order. Heal, get better, repair, renew or all of the above. I would rejuvenate my son's confidence simply by recovery.

I was determined to heal in the most efficient way possible. The best way forward was to pick wisely from the canteen menu (no more derision about hospital food from me). I was having any meal option that offered protein, whether I liked it or not. Any fish dish for lunch or egg product or yoghurt for breakfast, all washed down with tons of milk.

The essential building block for healing was protein so I ate omelettes that could have re-soled shoes. I had tuna mayo with so little mayo in it you'd need forensics to verify that an egg had ever been in the same room. I drank gallons of milk and still felt like Oliver; "Please sir, can I have some more?"

I longed for a bloody pizza but unless Dominos delivered an egg, anchovy and peanut pizza, I wasn't having it. My lower left drain was still putting out about six hundred millilitres of fluid a day (that's quite a lot of lymph, so I was told). The lower right stents were literally holding my kidneys and newly plumbed-in bladder together.

Healing needed to be well on the way before either of these tubes was removed. I was desperate to have them out as they were hindering my every movement. Only by building myself up, protein block by protein block, would I be free of these limiting bags.

Within a couple of days I was up and mobile again. A much needed shower was a delight. A convenient shower chair was installed and it was simple to gather all my tubes, shuffle across and set the water to "scald." Lee Child's fictional character Jack Reacher and I are absolute opposites in (almost) every conceivable way.

He's 6'5" and I'm 5'9" (if you stretch me out on the floor). He's a Military Policeman and I failed the draft. He's a master tactician and I struggle with joined-up writing. There are two aspects in common with Reacher that give me a kinship with the figure; a chemical dependency on caffeine and a deep love of hot showers.

Every day, sometimes twice a day, I would gather my baggage and shuffle into the stall. I would set the temperature as high as I could tolerate and stay there for a very long time. I was worried about Gartnavel's water bill.

I would sit for an age and let the water play over my newly sewn belly. It helped with the pain and discomfort. It was relaxing and restorative. In one of the fictitious Reacher books he suffers a disfiguring stomach scar which takes months to heal. That now makes three things in common.

Mr Crooks' daily visits were most often in the afternoons, after visiting was over. He was particularly interested in the post op drains. They were putting out large quantities of lymph. He had daily samples sent for analysis to rule out infection and we waited to see if the production would slow. I wouldn't be allowed home until it stopped. I willed it to heal over. I seriously wanted out.

The morning of the 20th February my routine started as normal. Awake by 6.30am, ask for some towels, head for the shower and be out in time for breakfast at half past seven. I looked forward to the shower every morning. It was a perfect wake up. I gathered my belongings and headed through to the en-suite. Careful to plonk the drains and stents on my lap, I transferred over into the cubicle.

There was a tearing sound and an almighty shooting pain in my right hip.

The tubes had caught under the wheelchair.

I had ripped the stents right out of my kidneys.

Taking the Piss

There was a pull-cord alarm in the cubicle; ostensibly for those with a fall risk on wet floors. I pulled the thing hard enough to yank it from the ceiling. I looked down but couldn't believe what I'd just done. I had the urinary bag on my lap alright. It trailed onto the floor, around the front right wheelchair castor and back up into my groin. I'd used the full dead-weight of the chair to wrench the stitches holding the stents in place.

What had I just done? Had I just ruined everything out of sheer stupidity? I was looking at two fine white tubes about fifty centimetres long. One was fully out. The other had less exposed length but not by much. There was very little residual pain but the idea that I had torn all the structures beneath was filling me with dread. I sat waiting for assistance and the "What Ifs?" started in my brain.

What if I've damaged the kidneys? What if I've torn the new bladder? What if they need to fix me all over again? What if there's not enough left intact to repair? What If they have to undo Mr Hendry and Simon's stitches? Perhaps they should just install a zipper or Velcro. The idea of another big procedure, judging by damage I'd caused, was harrowing.

One of the male nurses, David, came to assist. He taped the residual stent in place and we did a double transfer, first to the chair, then the bed. Barbara was next through the door and she sympathetic and consoling and assured me it was all going to be fine.

I was a bit shell shocked and didn't say much of anything. I was disproportionately calm about the whole situation. The dehisced stomach had far more gore and had been visually alarming but this was now potentially disastrous. I wasn't panicking wildly or falling away from reality. I simply stared at the two tubes hanging from their source. Barbara then said something that made my blood turn to ice.

"I'll see if we can get a hold of Mr Palmer."

Oh crap! He's going to be as mad as hell. I've screwed up big time and ruined some serious work. I don't know why I was so worried about what he'd say but I was suddenly terrified of his wrath. Not once had Mr Palmer given me the impression that he was an ogre but his opinion of what I had done to his skilful craft mattered mightily. Only once before had I felt like this.

At seventeen I had a provisional driving licence. My mate Gavin had one also. I had a car already waiting on me passing my test, which wasn't too far off. Gavin and I had an empty house and figured that two "provisionals" would make at least one full licence. We took the car out for a spin. We took it just around the block and back; not too far. It was highly irresponsible but at seventeen these things seem trivial even though they're deadly serious.

We brought it back to Dad's garage and Eddie was there in the empty space, pointing at me then to the space at his feet. I could feel the blood drain from my face. His eyes bored into mine. I could hear my heart beating in my ears. I had fucked up royally and was about receive the mother of all bollockings.

The memory of the event still sends shock waves through my psyche and waiting on Mr Palmer made my brain twitch the same way. I used the time to berate myself thoroughly. You total knob! How could you? Utterly useless arsehole! Careless, idiotic moron! You are a clown of epic proportions! You're so dense that light bends around you! (Malcolm Tucker quote again) Mr Palmer had arrived and interrupted my mental censure.

"I'm so sorry boss. It was an accident." I waited for the hammer to fall.

"Why are you sorry? These have probably been in long enough to have done the job. Why don't we just take all this out now? We'll leave you a couple of hours and see if the neo-bladder takes over."

He was extremely reassuring and supportive. He took the time to explain the stents placements and function. They were temporarily placed to stop post op swelling closing over the kidney's ureters. I f I hadn't made the mistake of ripping them out, they would have been removed soon anyway.

Where on earth had I got the impression he'd be mad? I could have kissed him. I may well have kissed him but his moustache would have tickled and I don't like tickly kisses. The nurse cleaned and dressed the hole where the stents had been and he said they'd be back later.

Time ground to a halt. I fretted like a madman. This was it. This was the summation of the surgery, the anaesthetic, the multiple pauses, the temporary pacemaker, the permanent pacemaker, the stress I heaped on my wife, family and friend all wrapped up in a desperate unspoken plea for pee.

I drank water like a man in the desert. I watched the clock, willing the time to speed up and get him back to see if things were working. I couldn't concentrate on books, TV, movies or music. Nurses popped in periodically to check I was ok. Of course I wasn't bloody ok. I needed to know now. Was the new plumbing intact?

At last he was here with the nurse and gloves and a foil bowl. "Shall we?"

Yes let's crack on! My brain was screaming inside. He was going to use a catheter to tap into the bladder and see if the kidneys had used the new setup. My fingers were crossed. My toes would have been crossed if I could use them. I watched Mr Palmer's every move, waiting for the "golden" moment.

Time slowed. I watched and watched and watched. A sudden jet of fluid hit the bowl and didn't stop. It was a glorious golden stream of piss. It kept coming and coming and coming. I smiled like the Cheshire cat. Job done; it was the perfect result.

He said "Happy?"

"Very! Thanks boss."

He and the nurse tidied up and before he left he asked,

"Paul, do you do the lottery?"

"No Mr Palmer."

"Good. I wouldn't if I were you. Not with your luck."

I laughed.

New Highs to New Lows

I revelled in my new freedom. The stents had been more limiting than the drain. One down, one more to go, then I'd be heading home. Stephanie and I could see the light at the end of the tunnel. Her commute to Gartnavel was long one. Factor in a full day's work and two kids to run after, plus the stress of me phoning with a new emergency every few days.

This girl had a tough life. Healing would continue for months after discharge but the sooner the drain stopped, the sooner I could be under my own roof and back with the family.

I was on a new drug regime to improve my blood chemistry. I was on sodium bicarbonate to regulate acidity levels. I was low on magnesium so required a supplement. I had various anti-inflammatory meds and pain killers to boot. I needed daily anti-coagulant injections to prevent a fatal clot. I'd take just about anything that was prescribed, just as long as it helped me heal and get home. I was three days into my new regime when I took very ill.

At first I thought it was just a dodgy tummy; all acidic and gurgling. Then I was violently sick and my guts ran through before I could get close to the toilet. I called for assistance and needed to be helped into the shower to clean off.

I was suddenly very weak and nauseous. I was shaking

violently. It didn't stop. My insides continued to pour out. It came in waves. It would be twisting cramps then terrible diarrhoea. It went on for hours. The doctors had no idea what was causing it.

Urgent blood work was ordered up. Was this infection? I had been open to the elements just days before. It was conceivable that a "nasty" had got into the wound and had set up camp. If not that, then what else could it be? Don't let it be the dreaded MRSA. That's a tough fight and would mean a very long stay in isolation to prevent it spreading. Anything but that.

I was now so weak I had to be lifted to and from the toilet and shower. Drips were put up to replace vital fluids that I was rapidly losing. I was so thoroughly done in, I could barely move. Where would this all end?

I had lurched from plight to predicament to dilemma and there was no end in sight. Just when things had become rosy again, I was back in danger. I was struggling to hang on again and no one knew why.

Staying conscious took effort. I would drift off from time to time and be completely unaware that I'd just been sick or the bed was again being changed. Nightmares were vivid and fever took over. Shivering and sweating and sick and weak, the next few hours were torture. To have made it this far, after all that had gone wrong and been put right, I didn't want to go out in a sweaty, shivering, shitty mess.

I couldn't get my head around the fact that yet another "something" was wrong. I found it hard to stave off catastrophic thoughts. I had plummeted off a mental cliff and no amount of faux-psycho techniques involving the kids were working. I wanted an end to all of this.

No one else factored into my thinking at this point. I simply wanted to be put to sleep like the dying dog I was. Another day in anguish would be a day to long. I squeezed my eyes shut tight and for the first time since I was a child, I prayed.

"God?"

"Are you there?"

"It's me, Paul."

"Can you do me a favour? I know I keep on denying you. I know, OK? Listen just for a second. I don't ever ask you for anything. I know it's coz I'm an atheist and all, but if your there, actually really there, you really have to help me out here. Just once! It's only one wee thing. It'll be my one and only request from you, I promise."

"Kill me."

"It's easy! Plane loads of your devotees die every day. Just let a brain vessel pop in my head. Or, give me a clot to the heart, anything. Stop all this, I can't take any more. It'll be easy. Just let me go, OK?"

"Can you hear me? Listen I know what you're going to say next."

"Don't worry about Stephanie. She's gorgeous and clever; she'll find someone else in no time. She deserves better than going through all this. Are you hearing me? Stephanie is a rock. She can move on with her life. And the kids are still young. It'll hurt them for only a little while. They'll forget it in time. They deserve more of a Dad than what's left of me. I can't go on any longer."

"God?"

"Are you listening, or what?"

"Fine, I'll even beg you. Please, please kill me. Please? Do it!"

"Can you hear me? Are you even there? If you're not there, that's one thing. You obviously can't help if you're a figment of the imagination. If you are there, that's another thing entirely.

If you are actually there and you can hear me then you're refusing to help. If that's the case and you refuse to help me this one time, well then…"

"Fuck you!"

"I'll do it myself."

I reached for the anti-coagulant in its pack, broke the seal and exposed the needle. Inject it into the neck and the brain haemorrhage would be inevitable and thankfully quick. I had just managed to get the tip into my carotid.

I woke up gasping, stunned and drenched in sweat. It was barely sunrise and the nightmare had seemed more real than the room around me. I actually felt my neck for blood. This was ridiculous. It had just been a fevered night terror. I was crushed by disappointment.

Not disappointed that I was still alive. It was because I had let myself down in any number of ways. I'd begged a deity, ignored the suffering of my wife and kids and subconsciously at least considered taking the easy way out. I was angry at myself.

"Anger is a gift" (Zack de la Rocha from the band RATM)

I'd now had enough of this mewling weakness and tapped into the anger I was feeling towards myself. At my weakest point I had considered the easy way out. I put some headphones on and deliberately selected the loudest, angriest track I have in my phone.

It's by the band Slipknot and is the perfect personification of wounded frustration, directed at the self.

I push my fingers into my eyes,

It's the only way that slowly stops the ache.

But it's made of all the things I have to take.

Jesus, it never ends.

It pushes way inside.

If this pain goes on, *I'm not gonna make it!*

(Duality by Slipknot)

The song is all noise and fury and naked aggression. I was incensed by my weakness. I reproached myself with the music still blaring in my ears.

How dare you give up on them? They deserve a better man. She's the goddess and you're letting her down. You are not worthy of your daughter's love. Your son idolises you. You are a weak, petty, small and pathetic excuse for a man.

The atavistic side of my brain chuckled to itself:

"See? You're a big girl's blouse."

To the Ultimate High

Barbara was a thing of beauty; her anger a great scourge and hugely entertaining to behold. She had come to my rescue and solved the latest problem.

Magnesium Sulphate is a supplement intended to replenish low levels of the mineral in the bloodstream. Magnesium Hydroxide is a powerful laxative that forms milk of magnesia when diluted in water. Guess which I had been given?

Barbara had found the error and was scything a path and "pointing out" what the consequences could have been. Once my prescription had been stopped, I rallied round quickly and thoroughly enjoyed the fireworks. If she had been attentive before, she was positively motherly now.

I couldn't have cared less where the error came from. I try never to play the blame game. And let's be honest, on checks and balance, my NHS had done more for me in this short time than against. The fact that I had made it this far was nothing short of a miracle (a miracle based on modern medicine, clinical expertise and quality nursing care). I was bouncing back after yet another close call and the overwhelming emotion was relief, not anger.

My self-imposed angry rebuke was also waning. I had now been using Tramadol as pain relief for days and its side effects were explained to me. It's a morphine derivative and amongst many other interesting things, causes night-sweats and night-mares. My emotional trough could easily be explained away by dehydration and altered brain chemistry. I could put a stop to the self-inflicted psychological beating for weakness.

I had a choice to either reduce my Tramadol intake and suffer greater pain or accept that my fevered mind might do some freaky gymnastics at night. As I was in such high levels of discomfort (unsurprisingly), I kept up with the current levels of pain relief. Once I got home I would kick these pills for sure. I resolved to be less harsh on myself if I developed sudden urges to join Scientology.

Food was staying down over the next couple of days. I was more comfortable and had entertainment at my fingertips. The steady streams of visitors were happy because I was more like myself. No more low-mood or self-flagellation. Night terrors were still happening but I was aware what was causing them, so forewarned was forearmed.

Moving around again meant I could build up some much needed muscle tone. I was fading away fast. My crash diet would ultimately drop my weight by a stone and a half. I wouldn't recommend this way to anyone else though; a slimming club was probably safer.

Mobility was also supposed to help the post op drains slow down. This was the next milestone. If they didn't begin to reduce their output, Mr Crooks was aiming to pull them out slightly. His theory was that the drain position may be resting on some lymph nodes, preventing them from healing. If that was the case, the drain was self-propagating. I was happy to have him try anything if it meant the end to tubes and bags.

Mum and Dad had not long left from their afternoon visit when Mr Crooks and Mr Rajan arrived. "Here we go" ran through my mind. Get the drain tugged back by a couple of inches and things may finally heal over. I would have no drains, catheters, pace leads or drips for the first time in weeks. I was looking forward to this like Christmas. I beamed a big hello to the two of them.

Mr Rajan closed the door and they both stood at the foot of the bed. There was no sign of gloves or stitch cutters or sterile drapes. They were here for something else. They were here for *the* something else. I was about to get my news. They were here as a double team to deliver *news!* My mind crashed about me.

"Oh shit no! I'm getting *bad* news. You always take another person along as a witness if it's bad news. Even I've done that before. Ah fuck! It must have spread everywhere! They took so long to tell me 'coz I was so ill. Now because I'm stronger they're able to drop the bomb. I'm here on my own! Surely I should have someone with me? Could they not wait till I have Stephanie here?"

I had a sudden flashback to Steven, his brother and girl-friend it was suddenly a blessing not to have anyone here. I'm not sure I could have mustered that guy's level of calm bravery. Let's just get this news done and over with and I'd deal with the fallout later.

My mouth was as dry as sand. My face prickled as though I'd developed a palsy. I could hear my pulse like a raging torrent in my ears. I'm sure my heart would have stopped if not for the pacemaker. My hands were shaking all on their own.

"Your histology results were posted this morning." Mr Crooks began.

"Sorry it took so long but they were just trying to make sure."

Months of pain, sweat and tears were distilled down into this moment. Fear, sickness, stress and effort was all for nothing if the cancer had spread. Could I continue on this journey?

I wasn't sure if I could take anything else after what had gone on. After all that had happened I was fairly sure I'd be refusing more treatment. I was fragile in psychology and physiology. If I were to forgo more treatment would my wife and family understand? Restarting chemo would crush me, I just knew it. No one ever discussed what would happen if the surgery was ineffective. Were there any treatments left? What if this is was my "limited" conversation, right here and now? How did Steven hold his nerve at this moment? I was sure I was about to vomit.

(No, no, no, no, no, no, no, no) My mind was screaming at me, trying to erect mental barriers for what was coming.

"All of your samples came back negative. There was no spread into the surrounding tissues."

(No, no, no, no. What?) I did a cartoon double take from Mr Crooks to Mr Rajan to Mr Crooks again. He went on.

"Before we get ahead of ourselves, you're not completely off the hook yet. There's no absolute guarantee that it can't come back. You'll receive six monthly scans to check progress. Otherwise for the immediate future it all went as well as could be expected."

He went silent. Mr Rajan was smiling. I was looking back and forth still not processing the good news.

"Thank you Mr Crooks." was all I could come up with.

I was taking my cue from his expression. Don't get ahead of yourself. It was good news but with a caveat. Don't celebrate just yet. No giddiness or high fives and shoulder charges. Just keep a lid on. Be the professional he expects you to be.

"I'll have one of the nurses retract that drain a little and see if we can't slow the output." He turned to go.

"Thanks again Boss."

As speeches go it sucked big-time. This crack team of professionals had saved me. My NHS had delivered me from the abyss. They had given me a future. They'd provided me with a quality of life that other cancer sufferers only dream of. I could have, should have expressed myself in any number of sincere ways.

Scores of unseen professionals had contributed to my care and would never know the impact they had on my life. What about the Biomedical Scientists or Pathologists who spent weeks pouring over my histology? He, she, they would never share in the joy of my good fortune.

What about the Radiologists or their Consultant who reported on my CT scans? He, she wouldn't get the job satisfaction of putting my delighted grin to the cold faceless 3D computer rendering. Did they all know how much it meant to me? Probably not.

The NHS employs 1.358 million staff and healthcare science comprises just five per cent of the total. Not even a significant minority, in numerical terms. Yet eighty five per cent of all medical diagnoses have healthcare science involvement. They are a small contingent with a huge significance.

Nurses are quite rightly the face of the modern NHS. Directly involved with patient care, they are huge in number and highly visible. Scratch the surface though and layer upon layer of unseen specialists were there contributing to my successful outcome. My thanks should have been better.

Thanks for the team effort to get me here. I'm indebted for your expertise in complex surgery. Thanks from my kids in still having a Dad who's coming home. Thanks from my wife in still having a husband at the end of all this. Thanks from all of my family and my true friend. That's what I should have said.

I could have said it in any one of a dozen profound and heartfelt ways to the man who epitomised the entire team. But me? In my shock and awe at the good news I could only muster,

"Thanks again Boss."

What a total dickhead!

Breaking News (the best kind)

"I wish I was a messenger. And all the news was good."

This is a memorable line from "Wishlist" by Pearl Jam. How good would that job be? To be a messenger with nothing but good news was how I felt after the doctors had gone. But I had a difficult choice.

Stephanie had to know first. She deserved to know before anyone else. After the journey she'd been through, it was only right. But do I phone right away or wait till she visited later that evening? Would I even be able to hold off? I could perhaps get her before she left work. If not, I'd have to wait for her to collect the kids. Then they'd be eating dinner in a hurry to get back out the door to make the journey to me in Gartnavel.

Since Mr Crooks' departure my chest was fit to burst with the news. I had to tell *someone*? No! Just wait and keep it to yourself. To stall her in any part of the packed schedule before visiting just delayed her from me. It was best to wait and do it in person.

I spent the time until evening visits considering my path to this point. I had an all clear, for the moment. The distant future was still unknown but the short to medium term was assured. I should have been on an indefatigable high but I had guilt nagging at my consciousness. This wasn't as acute as survivor's guilt. But bearing witness to an end of life conversation early on, I was aware that my fortune was not being shared by others just a short distance away.

No one could claim I'd had an easy time of it but some cancer fights were going on just as difficult, just as traumatic and without a silver lining like mine. It kept my mood stable, sober. Happy all the same but to revel in a successful outcome would be an insult to someone like Steven; a man perhaps half my age with twice the strength. I wouldn't ever wish to repeat my experience but I was content that the end justified the means.

The rollercoaster ride we had all been on was making its final turn and my family, my friend and I could at last climb off. From diagnosis to this point had taken eight months. Every conceivable emotion had been experienced by all. The overwhelming memories of the terror and the trauma would dull and fade with time. Normality, blessed routine and mundane events would soon occupy our day to day lives.

"All those moments will be lost in time. Like tears in the rain." (Roy's final words to Deckard in Ridley Scott's Blade Runner)

Evening meal came; I ate and hardly noticed that I'd done it. I was thoughtful. Not elated nor depressed. Just aware that I was thinking of a future for the first time where previously I hadn't. I wasn't conscious of limiting my viewpoint during the treatment but looking back I must had been. I had lived and thought only of the "here" and "now." It was a form of self-defence for the mind but suddenly I was thinking of "when" in the future tense.

Stephanie, Arianne and Jonathan arrived for the evening visit. This was it! I get to deliver *our* news! Right from the very start it had always been "our" or "we" when it came to dealing with cancer.

The people closest to you have just as hard a time. They have the helplessness and fear and guilt and stress which are magnified many times over when someone they love is critically ill. It's a team game when you are loved by this many. I was now getting to deliver the information that made it all worthwhile.

I let them get settled in and put the phone on for the kids to watch.

"Mr Crooks came by today." That wasn't ground breaking as he was checking on me almost daily.

"Hmm, what was he saying?"

Big deep breath and let's change her day.

"We got the all clear. It's all Ok. The histology was cancer free."

One one-thousand, two one-thousand, three one-thousand. Three seconds and the tears came. Stephanie grabbed my face in both hands and gave me a huge kiss then we hugged like we'd never let go. That started me off too, I couldn't help it. The relief was immense. We stayed like that for a long time.

We broke free and I recounted blow-by-blow the visit from the Consultant. Suddenly Arianne broke down and wailed,

"Can we *please* stop talking about Dad dying now?"

That stopped our conversation in its tracks. It was a heart-breaking moment. Ari had always seemed so upbeat and unaffected but her reality had obviously been very different. Months of hushed conversations and overheard phone calls had sunk in. Her Mum's stress must have been palpable. Her grandparent's fear and worry were poorly disguised. She had been slowly absorbing other's stress and doing a good job of hiding it from the adults.

She got pulled into a huddle with Jonny and Stephanie. I promised that the worst was over now. We all had the sort of release we'd sorely needed for weeks if not months. I was holding onto my family knowing, at last, I'd be around for some time to come.

The kids went back to the phone once we'd all calmed down. Stephanie and I planned for my future homecoming. All that was required for a clean getaway was for the drain to stop producing. One last barrier and I could spend the rest of my recovery convalescing under my own roof. This was a goal to work towards.

Visiting ended with massive hugs, kisses all round and lots of smiles. This would be the turning for the better and the news needed to be shared farther afield. I phoned my nearest and dearest and exchanged yet more misty eyed moments with them. Such good news was well overdue for all of them and delivering it made me feel like Santa for grown-ups. I was truly a messenger and the news was very, very good.

The most significant day came to an end. Emotionally drained but extremely happy, I could now let go of fear and worry and concentrate on strength and fitness. My crazy brain though, wasn't finished with me yet.

That night, the grim reaper tried to rip out my pacemaker. He was deeply angry that I had escaped so many times. My NHS had defied him and he was determined to finish the job personally. I went crashing through a darkened recovery ward looking for help but it was empty. Everyone had gone for the night.

I could sense him behind me as I was running away (I'm never, ever in a wheelchair in my dreams). I could feel his skeletal hand reach over my left shoulder, trying to tear out the device under my clavicle. Ducking and dodging, I narrowly avoided being caught but the drip stand I was dragging kept catching on corners.

I could feel him gaining. His breath was catching the hair on the back of my neck. The reaper caught the tie at the back

of my hospital gown and made a final grab for my collarbone.
I woke up gasping and sweaty.

Bloody Tramadol

Feeling Drained

Over the next couple of days I felt great. Apart from the stomach pain, the pacemaker discomfort, the carotid scar, the stent hole and the drain tube. It amazed me how a new perspective altered the sensations. Pain that previously would have taken serious will power to ignore, I now hardly felt.

The news was good.

I'd had the news, processed the news, shared the news and was now dealing with a new mental itch. Let's get out of here. Let's get home. Let's get better. Let's get back to work. My brain was getting way ahead of itself. The spirit is willing but the flesh was still very weak

The drain tube was still putting out a consistent five hundred millilitres per day. It was the remaining limitation to getting out and still a damned nuisance to move around with. Unless it started to slow down I'd be stuck here indefinitely.

I had been charting my own fluid balances, so I knew exactly what was draining away. I had also been swapping my own dressings on the now vacated catheter site and injecting my daily anti-coagulant. Anything to help, plus I like feeling involved. The bit I couldn't do for myself came next.

One of the nurses came with a sterile tray. She exposed the drain tube which was as thick as my index finger. She proceeded to remove the stitches holding it to my left hip and gave it a gentle pull. It stayed firmly put. A little light sprinkle of sterile water and she tried another pull. Nope, it didn't budge an inch.

We shared an ironic smile. She rolled her shoulders as though she was about to dead-lift a bar bell. This time it was a sharp tug. My hips move slightly toward her, still not good enough. I could see frustration building on her brow.

Now standing over me, left hand flat on my hip and right hand around the tube, she looked like she was about to start an outboard motor. She pulled and pulled and pulled some more. There was no real pain but it did feel like someone pulling wildly at your belly through a letter box.

There was a sudden smacking sound like a wet cloth dropped on tiles. The tube gave by about four inches. My nurse looked more relieved than I did. The only way of holding it in place without re-stitching was to tape it down. A bunch of tape and some fresh dressings and that was me back in order. Fingers crossed that this would have the desired effect.

I moved about as much as I was able. Activity was supposed to help the lymph nodes heal, so I got up out of bed for the majority of each successive day. Only when I got truly exhausted or particularly pained did I relent and lie down.

Within twenty four hours the improvement was obvious. Output was halved. Just as Mr Crooks had predicted, the drain tube was preventing healing. If it continued this trend, discharge from the ward was assured.

I was comfortable, well fed and entertained. Top Gear had started a new series and I could watch on the BBC catch up service. I was a thoroughly happy bunny. I turned the self-indulgence dial to eleven; reading, watching, listening and eating all my favourite things. The itch never really went away though. Let's get outa Dodge. At the first sign of recuperation I wanted to resume my old routine as if I were the same man.

Dawn's first actual visit since the good news was a welcome one. A great big hug and we were smiles all round.

"Well, what did I tell you?"

She had every right to be pleased with herself. Positivity had won the day. Her prediction had come true and the battle, if not the war, was over. She had just finished a shift at the Royal and headed straight to the ward in Gartnavel. This had the effect of her visit coinciding with meal time. Visiting during dinner in the ward was strictly forbidden.

Breakfast, lunch and dinner times in a ward are a hive of furious activity. All the staff are shuttle running back-and-forth to rooms with plates, drinks, cutlery, trays, you name it. Any interruption is most unwelcome. Factor in problems like an absence of someone's food order or someone having changed their mind without telling. It slows the whole process down and staggers meals into actual visiting.

Dawn had just casually strolled into the ward like any other member of the NHS. She was wearing her scrubs, so could have any one of a hundred valid reasons for being there. Visiting her pal was not a valid reason.

She was sitting on the high backed visitor chair, shoes off with her feet on my bed when Barbara walked in with my tray. Uh-oh, she's going to get tossed out on her ear by the boss, was my thinking.

"Barbara, this is Dawn. She and I work together at the Royal." Keep it light Paul and she might get away with a telling off. It might work but Barbara was not to be messed with.

"Hello Dawn, lovely to meet you." I was waiting for the stern telling off.

"Can I get you a spot of dinner? Shall I see if we have anything going spare?"

When she'd gone, we burst out laughing. Barbara really was looking out for me in a big way.

We sat with our food and talked about the world; the department, my ward, the histology, Stephanie, the kids. We covered it all. It made me itch all the more to get out as soon as possible. The world was still going on without me! How dare it!

It was all the more frustrating to know that even when I did get home to Stephanie and the kids, I still had roughly twelve weeks before I could get back to work. Escaping the ward was only the beginning. I had a lot of healing left to do.

Forty eight hours later the drain dried up.

Escape from Alcatraz

Alcatraz is being disingenuous. I'd had nothing but great care and attention in Gartnavel. But seeing the world through a window is still not the same as being part of it. I had become single-minded. I wanted to go home! As fun as it first felt, I couldn't fill all day, every day with books and movies. Over indulgence was making me sick.

The last few days of February were glorious. The weather was dry and crisp. Just the kind of day Stephanie and I would take the kids round the park for long walks. Then as a reward we would have a sweet snack and hot drinks in a café somewhere. I intrinsically knew those days were a long way off but to be mobile again and see more than four walls was the plan.

The drain removal was almost an ant-climax. Once it had stopped producing, it positively fell out of its own accord. The nurse who took it out was done before I had realised she'd started. The tape removal was the hardest part. The drain needed no coaxing to pull free. It positively slipped out of its own accord. This was the easiest procedure I'd been through by a long margin.

Unencumbered, I was truly mobile again. I could trundle up and down the ward fetching my own towels. I could hop on and off the shower seat with no compunction. I could wear clothes! Real boy clothes, not hospital gowns tucked strategically to avoid showing visitors my arse.

The new found freedom had an oddly negative effect. Moving around began to feel like the pacing up and down of a caged animal. The feeling of incarceration wasn't helped by the chain link on the windows. I knew it was to stop roosting birds but from the inside it really did begin to feel like prison bars.

The difference to the perpetually dying bloke weeks before was remarkable. I had considered my mortality and the meaning of life. I had previously wondered if I had done enough with my life; helped others enough, loved my kids hard enough, told my parents I loved them enough, kissed my wife enough. None of this was being taken for granted but I was aching with the need to get out of hospital.

On the last Saturday in February I asked if I was allowed to go outside for some fresh air. I also knew from a friend in Audiology that extra clinics were in effect downstairs so decided to pay some friends a visit. I felt like Lazarus.

The greetings were raucous. The shocked faces were hilarious. The stunned faces at the good news were even more hilarious. They weren't as hilarious as the horrified faces when I showed them the picture of my stomach wound. I now had a party piece to trump all others. I was keeping that picture forever, just in case I wanted to scare small children.

I spent a half hour then let them get back to their clinic and took my book and a double espresso outside. I couldn't believe this was winter. The trees were bare. Grit salt had been spread by a pessimistic council but there wasn't a cloud in the sky. The sun was strong enough to be warm. There was not a breath of wind. It was a glorious day to be out and about.

I parked up next to a bench and put my coffee on the seat. I pulled out my Samsung and navigated to the latest Jack Reacher novel. Another patient appeared with a drip stand and virtually collapsed onto the seat next to me. He rummaged around in his dressing gown pocket and came out with cigarettes and a lighter. He lit up and started puffing away.

The bench had a no smoking sign on it. The wall, the bin, the hospital sign and the concrete entrance all had signs on them.

"THE HOSPITAL GROUNDS ARE A NO SMOKING AREA."

After months being plagued with endless Gestapo-like questions regarding my smoking status, the irony was acute. I moved off. No way was I about to sit and absorb second hand smoke. I found a secluded patch of grass with a bus stop on one side and a glass wall on the other. This was even better, warmer too.

I had just found the paragraph where I had left off when a staff member arrived and promptly started smoking. Looking around, this was obviously a favourite hidey hole. Butts were strewn all around. I was pissed off now. I was here first! I glared at her. She tried hard to ignore me. I glowered at her harder. She deliberately avoided eye contact.

I made a teenager huffy noise and moved off again. I found a far-away bench, as far from the entrance as I could. Let's see someone drag their bloody drip this far out. No more than ten minutes passed when some young bloke sat down.

He pulled out a pack. No goddamn way. I was not for moving. Not again. I leaned in towards him and I whispered with all the menace I could muster.

"I've already moved twice to avoid smokers."

"If you take one of them out, I'm going to shove it so far up your arse, you'll have to set fire to your nose to light it."

I delivered it flat, deadpan. I clearly wasn't kidding. It was actually a verbatim quote from the movie Heartbreak, Ridge made by the legend Clint Eastwood. The young guy put the pack back in his pocket, stood up and moved off towards the entrance to be with the rest of his kind.

I was totally relieved. He fell for it! He could have knocked me over with a huff and a puff. I was as weak as a day old kitten and had nothing to back it up with. I settled down for a good hour of reading and caffeine and felt very pleased with myself.

I recounted my cheeky comment to Stephanie at visiting that night. I'm not too sure she approved. We were both lying cuddled up on the hospital bed. This would definitely be frowned upon if someone came in, but who cares? With no tubes coming out of me I could lie on either side. Or lie close to the lady in my life. It was a slice of normality and a sign of better things to come.

Ward rounds the following morning were a very relaxed affair. It was Sunday and rather than being early o'clock, it was mid-morning before a threesome of doctors showed up.

Bloods had been taken every day for a month and things were returning to normal. They were all very happy with the new stomach repair (none more so than I). The high tensile sutures would be taken out in a few weeks' time by community nurses. The dressings were fresh and shower-proof. The pacemaker was on-song and worth its weight in gold. All-in-all I was thoroughly on the mend.

"You seem to be very self-sufficient," The lead doctor said; which was true. I preferred to just get on with my own dressings and meds and allow the staff to deal with the other patients.

"I don't see any reason why we shouldn't let you home."

"What today?" This seemed too good to be true. It was a wish come true.

"You'll need some pharmaceuticals before you leave but these shouldn't take more than an hour to order."

"Thank you *very* much." I had a Cheshire cat grin a mile wide.

A hasty phone call to Stephanie and I was packing up like a removals man. I had accumulated a ton of stuff; books, magazines, several changes of clothes, cards, toiletries and food. So much food in fact, I'm sure that some of the visitors thought ten thousand calories per day were still not enough.

My prescriptions took slightly longer than an hour and came in a carrier bag. I had dressings and tubes and medicines and wipes and gloves. It was enough to resupply a cottage hospital. There was stuff I had never seen before and had never used. Not one to argue, I shut up about it and maintained my gratitude at escaping.

Stephanie was still a good hour out but I decided I'd wait for her at the front. It was another glorious day (actually and metaphorically) so I asked if I could leave and wait outside. I bid my farewells.

The ward had taken excellent care of me despite my multiple attempts to undo their hard work. There were lots of "Stay out of trouble" type comments from everyone. Barbara was sadly absent as she had her days off. I tried to be as effusive in my thanks as possible but thanks seemed a bit weak. Considering what had been done to / for me, I owed a bit more than words.

Stephanie and the kids pulled up two hours after the doctor had mentioned "home" and I was never so happy to see them. They had come in my Suzuki jeep as her car was totally unsuitable (a low two door coupe sporty thing). I gingerly hoist myself up into the passenger seat and Stephanie stowed the chair and luggage in the back.

We set off up Great Western Road, the road so often travelled in the past few weeks. It was catharsis to be making it one last time. I was finally heading home after jumping from the frying pan, into the fire, into the abyss and back out again, repeatedly. Home meant rest, recuperate and the comfort of my own bed.

I was wrong again.

Tramadol Nights

Moving around our home that afternoon felt very odd. Everything was familiar enough. Stephanie had soup readied in the slow cooker. The fruit bowl was overflowing. Remote controls were scattered about the living room. Kid's toys were piled up at the bottom of the stairs. The bed was made with its customary twenty two pillows (two pillows to put your head on, the other twenty for decoration).

I felt completely out of place. When we return from holiday the house always feels cold and inert. We then heat and invigorate it with our presence and make it a home again. This day, it was already active and full and alive. I felt as if I were an interloper. It didn't feel quite like mine. It should have, all the bills for it come out of my wage!

Stephanie watched me like a hawk for the rest of that day. I wobbled up and down to and from the couch. I trundled around the kitchen. Every time I was out of sight for more than sixty seconds she would ask if I was ok. It was one thing to want your husband home. But in having him home, he was suddenly very vulnerable if something unexpectedly went wrong. There was no medical backup at the end of a call button now. I had built up a bit of a reputation in the preceding weeks.

We enjoyed a family Sunday dinner. It was manna from heaven and completely surreal after the dramatic five weeks.

The evening was taken up with phoning family to let them know I was home. The kids had a traditional early Sunday bed in preparation for school the following day and I wasn't that far behind them. Some evening TV and a cuddle on the couch: that was the first day of freedom done and dusted; bed time.

Everyone thinks that *their* bed is the most comfortable bed in the whole world. It's what people comment about when they return from holiday. "Ahh there's nothing as comfortable as your own bed." But they're wrong, all of them. *My* bed is the most comfortable bed in the whole world, especially that night. But it didn't last.

Within two days I couldn't rest. I couldn't sleep. I couldn't stop shaking and sweating. I looked like a Parkinson's sufferer. My legs moved rhythmically like I was pedalling an imaginary bicycle. My hands shook like an alcoholic with Delirium Tremens.

Tramadol withdrawal

My initial joy at being home evaporated. I was a jittery wreck. I shook non-stop day and night. It had to be borne out though, if not now then at some future point. I couldn't bear the thought of postponing the inevitable. If I could just grit my teeth and bear it, I would kick these hugely addictive pain killers.

I researched others' methods online to see if there was a way to mitigate the side effects. There was no miracle solution to be had unfortunately. Most people's experiences were reminiscent of the scene in "Trainspotting" where Renton writhes on a bed during withdrawal. A great many people were significantly worse off having been on higher doses for much longer. The conservative estimate was I'd be suffering from ten to twenty one days.

And nights. The night times were hardest. After longing for the comfort of my own bed for weeks, I was unable to sleep in it. Even when I did manage to sleep the nightmares were vivid: drowning was a regular scenario as was the ever present chase by the Grim Reaper. To top it off were the muscle spasms. All night long my legs pulsed and the involuntary twitching kept Stephanie awake. I resigned myself to sleeping on the couch. Otherwise we'd both be up all night.

Moving around during the day kept the shakes to a controllable minimum but if I attempted anything requiring fine motor control, forget it. I dribbled fluids, food fell off my fork and playing on the Playstation became a joke.

My car on all driving games lurched from side to side. My coordination on strategy games was pathetic and Call of Duty was impossible. Playing online against some American kids, my soldier turned a virtual corner and caught one guy totally unawares, with his back to me.

My avatar pulled a rifle and emptied a whole magazine at him. I stitched a perfect outline and missed with every bloody bullet. The little git dropped me with one shot and laughed at me solidly for five minutes.

I abandoned the games console and stuck to TV and books. The problem was, unless the TV was Top Gear (or car related at the very least), I wasn't that interested. Books then; they had to be propped on a solid surface to allow me to read. My shaking was giving me nystagmus as my eyes had to keep tracking the moving text. Sod this for a laugh, how soon could I go back to work?

Not soon enough as far as I was concerned. I was still not allowed to drive. I still had a huge sensitive wound, tremors and weakness. Being housebound caused huge frustrations. The flesh was still weak but the spirit was willing and impatient and bored being stuck indoors.

Dawn continued to visit every week. She came to the house on her days off to check that I was actually resting and not over doing matters. She indulged me so that I could pretend with her that I still had a say in the departmental running. She was doing such a good job in my absence I was worried about going back. Was I going to step on her toes (in the absence of a wheelchair equivalent)? Was I now surplus to requirements?

It would be weeks before I was match fit. How rusty does any person get when they've been out of circulation for a fortnight's holiday? I know it takes me a couple of days to find my groove after just two weeks away. This was to be an absence six times longer. I was worried about going back, even this early on. I decided to contact the boss at Occupational Health.

I emailed Rona and gave her a summary of what had been going on. The reply was a couple of minutes later with the tag line: phone me! I duly did and a forty minute phone call ensued. She was surprised to say the least. Worry and concern were evident from the call. The suggestion she made that I extend my basic convalescence got shot down in flames.

Rona proffered the idea that I take as much time as necessary to get my physiology and psychology back to normal. I offered back that my physiology had never been anything to write home about (I was not about to be offered a modelling contract pre-surgery). That and my psychology would be best served with something to keep it occupied.

Counselling was offered and refused. There was concern, not just from her that I would have a period of post-traumatic stress. I arrogantly dismissed it outright. I only wished to know how quickly I could phase back into clinic once the majority of my physical wounds were healed. I'm sure Rona still thinks to this day that I'm nuts.

We had a few calls over the intervening weeks where she was conspicuously trying to gauge my mental health. She never gave up but I stuck to my assertion that the best way forward was routine. I had a second ulterior motive to returning: money.

I had used up my annual leave pre-surgery on the chemo days. I was now quickly getting through my paid sick leave. If I didn't get back to full time hours by early June my pay was at stake. Every day stuck at home meant one day closer to a fifty per cent cut in wages.

Others' assertion that it was "only money" conveniently forgot about car payments, mortgage, food, heat and light. All through treatment and in the darker days post-surgery I would think: what happens to Stephanie if I die? Could she afford to keep our kids in our home with her single wage? Have I enough life insurance to pay off the house? How would she manage?

Even on the mend, I considered that if I wasn't back to work in a flash, some of the home comforts may have to sacrificed. Satellite TV, mobile phones, gym membership, there were lots of cuts that could be made if I wasn't able to recover in the time frame that remained.

The best thing I could do was not screw up. To over-do matters and set my healing back would be inviting catastrophe. Frustrating it may well be, but if I had a time window in which to heal, doing something silly would be unforgivable. And potentially it would be financially ruinous. Patience was a virtue I was born without.

Things were definitely improving, even if they weren't improving at my preferred rate. Within two weeks it was obvious that the shaking was less. I was spending less time on the sofa under a blanket. I now could get in and out of the car unassisted. My strength was coming back, my beard was back and the party balloons in my undershorts had shrank back to normal size. To top it all off, the community nursing team were happy enough with the wound that the stitches could come out.

Hi-Ho, Hi-Ho.....

The community nurse was all set with the stitch cutters. I was lying back on my bed trying to feign indifference. Inside I was shitting myself. Flashbacks to my dehisced episode kept popping up in my brain. Won't happen this time, I kept telling myself. It might! Nah, not this time. BUT IT MIGHT! Shut up brain.

These damn stitches were indeed high tension. The poor nurse dug and dug. She snipped and cut and tweezered and then cut some more. It wasn't particularly comfortable but I had to just grit my teeth and allow her to crack on. She laboured down there for a very long time. She was gone so long in fact I was expecting her to come up with something rivalling the Bayeux Tapestry.

These weeks at home had altered me drastically. Food and rest had combined to see my colour return. Stephanie had previously driven us about but now I was allowed to drive. We'd had gentle days out and walked around various parks. I had deliberately kept my urges to strive and push in check. It was an exercise in self-control but had been worth it.

My nurse had finished. I gently sat up with assistance. Tentative movements got me to the 'chair. I thanked her profusely for the amount of time she spent and saw her to the door. Then I had a good poke and a prod at the unsupported tummy.

Success: all was well. I was just as secure without the sutures as with them. Healing was well and truly established. Rest, recuperation and Stephanie's excellent cooking had combined to knit the wound beautifully. A simple sterile dressing was all that was required to prevent my clothes rubbing against the wound.

Two weeks later it was off to work we go. Not yet in my professional guise but as an outpatient for a pacemaker check. I deliberately went to the Royal an hour early to visit my mates. It was a sort of homecoming: lots of hugs and kisses. A great many comments too about how well I looked. My cardiology appointment was at 1.30pm so I stayed with my lot for a spot of lunch then trundled up the corridor to the waiting room.

I'd barely got the phone out for a spot of reading when I was called through into a clinic room. The Cardiologist was a very pleasant lady and her space was a Glasgow Royal identikit room. A sink, a bed, kitchen-style units, wipe clean chairs and a truly awesome free-standing machine.

Her gear looked like something from the 50s Flash Gordon movies. It had a big display with a touch pen stylus, a keyboard with too many superfluous keys, an attached printer and wiring. There were dozens of multi-coloured wires coming out of it. They were all for me.

She wired me up in the traditional heart tracing way. Leads were attached to ankles, forearms and chest. Next a probe was draped around my shoulders and sited over the pacemaker. This looked like a big flat coaster with wiring which wound around me, along the floor and up to Flash Gordon's TV set.

The pacemaker and it communicated wirelessly with various parameters. It could tell how often it had paced. It recorded how my heart rate had been over the previous few weeks and it could even predict its remaining battery life.

The Cardiologist ran through a series of tests and graphs and print-outs just to confirm the device was working well.

"It all seems to be working fine. It's pacing about seventeen percent of the time and based on current levels, the battery should last another nine years."

I was quite happy with that. No need to change the device for nearly a decade seemed like a good result to me. However something was amiss.

"Hang on; there was a big anomaly eight days ago. Your heart rate spiked to a peak of 198 beats per minute. Were you unwell at any point?"

I thought back to last Tuesday but came up blank. I'd been feeling better and better with each passing day. Even the withdrawal period was becoming a dim memory. I definitely hadn't been unwell. Then something occurred to me.

"You know what, I remember now. It's all fine."

"It's not fine. That's very high." She clearly was expecting an explanation. Crap! How was I going to explain this without embarrassing either of us?

"Well, you see, well, it's just that we, I mean my wife and I were, you know checking to see if stuff worked." I even did air parenthesis with my fingers on the word "stuff." She didn't follow.

"I don't follow."

"Well, we were checking to see if stuff (air parenthesis again) worked after surgery. It does." She looked blank. I wasn't getting my point across well at all.

"Stuff! You know husband and wife stuff?"

The Cardiologist was now looking at me as if I was talking total gibberish. She soundlessly mouthed the word stuff to herself a couple of times. She's gonna make me say it, I thought. I'm actually going to have to say it out loud. I raised my eyebrows expectantly and waited a minute. The penny thankfully dropped.

"Oh? OH! OH I see!"

Yep, she saw and I smiled. What followed was the quickest tidy-up of wires you've ever seen. I had another appointment made for three months. Leaving the clinic, I wondered idly how many anomalies I could get showing on my trace before I was due back. That was a challenge worth taking on. OK pacemaker, get recording.

My carotid scars were well and truly healed. I'd had great fun picking the scab from the pacemaker site (why do we derive such pleasure from the masochistic re-opening of scar tissue – or maybe that's just me). The stomach was well on the way and at this point I was just a month from phasing back into work. My patience was screwed down tight. Time was my friend and haste would be my undoing.

With less than a fortnight to go an agreement was bartered out with Rona, Forbes and most importantly Stephanie. I would start by doing two days in the first week, three days the second week and so on. After a month had gone by I should theoretically be able to maintain full time hours. I would be making it back by the skin of my teeth, before full sick pay ran out.

Stephanie was both sceptical and supportive in equal measure. With a past history of pretending to be OK when I was anything but, she had every reason to be guarded. The twelve weeks convalescing at home had been frustrating, painful, boring but absolutely necessary. From the birthday in February to now it had been a journey from one milestone to the next.

At some points the milestones had been simply survive to the day's end. Other milestones were about climbing up and out of a psychological trough. The discharge from hospital had been a high point on the journey and months later the last barrier to normality was now just one sleep away.

Tomorrow I would don a uniform and go back to Dawn and my NHS.

Manchester II

Stephanie, the kids and I were spending a couple of days in Manchester. The plan was to take the kids to Alton Towers for a full day of thrills and spills. We were using the city as a staging post pre-theme park and had booked a cheap hotel to stay in. The weather was outstanding, the city centre was packed and Andy Murray had just started what would be the most memorable Wimbledon final since 1936.

Strolling around the city we came across The Shakespeare pub. Outside it the tennis final was being shown on a huge TV. Every available space was occupied with supporters of the Dunblane boy as he started the first set. It was a party atmosphere everywhere around us.

It was July and we were taking a short break in lieu of a holiday much later in the year. My health had improved markedly but it was suggested we not travel abroad for the first six months, just in case. The kids though still needed some sort of entertainment to look forward to, so a mini trip south would do the trick.

We came across the very same water fountain Stephanie had been pictured in. The weather was so very warm that the kids spent ages happily running through, getting drenched. Jonny had his arm's plaster cast covered in a carrier bag, having broken it badly falling off a climbing frame weeks prior.

What the hell is it with Doody men and hospitals? (Stephanie)

Manchester the year before had been a poignant pre-treatment pretence at normality. This year it was a family outing that felt comforting in its familiarity. The previous fear and loathing was replaced by fun and loving. The Radiohead concert and its mountain metaphor were long past and life had returned to a recognisable routine.

"But that place on Memory Lane you liked

Still looks the same but something about it's changed."

(Fireside by Arctic Monkeys)

The initial phase-in to work was highly amusing. I was welcomed into the fold like "Norm" from Cheers. The prodigal son was well and truly home. It took no time at all for the everyday work pressures to build up to the point that cancer was completely forgotten about.

I tried hard (and continue to try) not to undo Dawn's hard work in the department. My skill set had deteriorated drastically but necessity meant that I found my feet soon enough. The email in-box had to be seen to be believed. It took days to sift through it all but most if not all had been already actioned by Dawn many months before.

After only a few weeks back, perspectives were already being lost, just as I knew they would. Things that shouldn't matter, suddenly seemed deathly important. Minor stressors began to feel major.

The guy in the cardiac bed from February would have mocked the other who was supposedly stressed at his work. Memories became short. In looking back to normal you get treated as though you are back to normal: even if things couldn't be farther from the truth.

I wouldn't have it any other way. Keeping a record of events helps this. The main purpose in writing about my journey is to maintain the perspective between minor and major.

The perceived differences between the two Manchester's were huge both in temperature and feel. One was dark and cold, fearful and foreboding. The other was warm and bright, positive and joyous (helped in no small part by Mr Murray winning).

The second Manchester would not have been possible without your NHS.

Your NHS

It's your NHS and you shouldn't hear a bad word against it. In turns it has been my educator, my employer and now my saviour.

I couldn't possibly hope to pay back what I have used in resources from the NHS. It would take me another lifetime to pay forward the contributions: a lifetime that I don't have.

This lifetime, the one that was so nearly cut short, continues due to the on-going efforts of 1.358 million workers. It would be impossible to mention everyone involved in my care. The names alone could fill a phone book.

There were two shift patterns in every ward. Porters, domestic assistants, nurses, doctors, scientists of every discipline were involved in saving me and rescuing me from the abyss. Even greater scores of unseen, faceless professionals continue to save their fellow man day, after day, after day.

Not everyone is able to be saved though. Steven has most likely gone "wherever we might go" based on his consultation all those months ago. He and I shared only a few actual words one night but very different fates. His brother, girlfriend and I will only remember a fraction of what made the man whole: a shadow remains of the light that he shone.

Our outcomes were true opposites. His cancer won out, mine was repelled. I had my first of the six monthly CT results just two days ago: all clear. He was strong at the end for others, in a way that few of us could ever be. That's why the dedication at the beginning is to him.

These pages also serve as a long love letter to my NHS. You saved me and deserve so much more than just words.

But words will have to do.

Thanks to every last one of you,

from Stephanie, Arianne, Jonathan and Me.

x

Paul Doody BA, MPPM, RHAD

Professional Profile

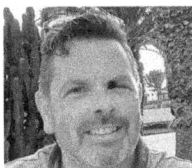

Chief Audiologist in the NHS

Specialist Tinnitus adviser

Queen Margaret University examiner and trainer.
[Audiology Bsc and MSc]

Tinnitus and Hyperacusis Master class

20th European Instructional course on
Tinnitus and Hypercusis.

Lightning Source UK Ltd.
Milton Keynes UK
UKHW040613100220
358470UK00013B/338

9 780993 483363